Micromethods for the Clinical and Biochemical Laboratory

Micromethods for the Clinical and Biochemical Laboratory

Hermann Mattenheimer, M. D.

Senior Biochemist
Presbyterian-St. Luke's Hospital
Chicago, Illinois

Professor of Biochemistry
College of Medicine
University of Illinois

aa
sp

ANN ARBOR ■ LONDON

ann arbor science publishers inc.

Drawer No. 1425. 600 S. Wagner Road, Ann Arbor, Michigan 48106

Berlin
Second edition 1966
Translated from the second edition by the author.

Library of Congress Catalog Card No. 71-96866
SBN 016-87591-5
Printed in the United States of America

Ann Arbor Science Publishers, Ltd.
5 Great Russell Street, London, W. C. 1, England

Foreword

In recent years there has been an avalanche of techniques and instruments available for the analysis of components of interest to the biochemist and clinical chemist. Each time a new technique is made known, numerous papers appear describing modifications to it, and the laboratory worker who desires to use these methods is faced with the difficult choice of which variant to use. Dr. Mattenheimer has performed a most useful service for us in this volume by describing in detail the instrumental and methodological requirements for proper microchemical analyses. The methods presented have been thoroughly tested and their reliability and accuracy proven by daily use. Even the busiest of laboratories will find these microliter methods advantageous for many of their high volume routine procedures. The obvious savings in time, space and money of micromethods are of concern to us all.

Max E. Rafelson, Jr., Ph.D.

John W. and Helen H. Watzek
Chairman of Biochemistry,
Presbyterian-St. Luke's Hospital
and
Professor of Biological Chemistry
University of Illinois
College of Medicine
Chicago, Illinois

Preface

About forty years ago the development of biochemical micro- and ultramicromethods began at Carlsberg Laboratory, Copenhagen. In the hands of Linderstrøm-Lang and H. Holter and their many co-workers and students, this new approach opened the way for biochemical studies on minute cell, tissue and fluid samples.

From 1955–57 I received my training in micromethodology in Dr. Holter's department at Carlsberg Laboratory. Although my research project was the enzymology of amoeba, my interest grew in the development of micromethods in clinical chemistry. Of the various approaches possible for the development of micromethods, I chose, whenever possible, the proportional reduction of sample and reagent volumes. In this way it was possible to convert widely accepted and well tested conventional macromethods into micromethods—or microliter methods, to use a more modern term. The application of micromethods to routine clinical chemistry had to await the commercial manufacture of the necessary special equipment, which is now available.

A limited collection of micromethods was published in the first German edition of this book in 1961. The wide acceptance and favorable reviews of the book led to the revised and substantially enlarged second German edition in 1966, which covers the almost complete line of chemical and enzymatic methods requested from a modern clinical laboratory.

The first American edition is a translation of the second German edition with only a few revisions necessitated by the differences in the market for equipment and reagents between Europe and this country. In addition a few of the methods have been substituted for procedures more commonly used in the United States. With a few exceptions the micromodifications described in this book were worked out in my laboratory. The methods that were originally published as micromethods are marked with *micromethod* behind the literature reference.

The content of this book is not limited to routine clinical chemistry but includes techniques for biochemical research with a special chapter on ultramicrotechniques, which were mainly developed by O. H. Lowry and are suitable to quantitatively measure enzyme activity in a few cells dissected from frozen-dried tissue sections.

The research in my laboratory is supported by grants from the United States Public Health Service.

Chicago, Illinois
April, 1970

Hermann Mattenheimer

Contents

Chapter 1

Micromethods: Definition and Experience

The term micromethod is ambiguous and can be used to describe several methods:

1. It refers to a method which detects a substance present in very small amounts in a relatively large volume. The prefix "micro" denotes the concentration. To detect the substance in question, either it must be enriched or extremely sensitive techniques must be employed.
2. It refers to a method which analyzes a small volume for a substance present in a relatively high concentration. The prefix "micro" denotes the volume. If the volume is between 10 μl and 100 μl (1 μl = 0.001 ml) the method is called a *microliter method,* a term introduced only recently. All analytical procedures in Chapters 4–7 of this book belong to this group of tests.
3. It refers to a method which analyzes a small volume for a substance present in a relatively low concentration. The prefix "micro" denotes the volume as well as the concentration. Depending on the size of the volume such a method may still be a microliter method, but with volumes of less than 10 μl, down to a fraction of a microliter, one speaks of an ultramicromethod (Chapter 8). For example, ultramicro analytical procedures include fluorometry.

The number and variety of tests have increased substantially during the past 15 years, and a request for five or more analyses on a single blood sample of a patient today is about an average figure. Most macromethods require 1 ml of serum, and for five tests done in duplicate this comes to 10 ml serum or 20 ml blood. Repeated withdrawal of such quantities, particularly from severely sick patients, often becomes undesirable.

Considering the number of tests performed on infants' blood it is not surprising that pediatricians urge the use of microliter methods. For microliter methods, the chemist needs at most one-tenth of the volume ordinarily required for macromethods; thus five or more tests can be performed on 1 ml of serum.

Microliter methods have several advantages for the routine clinical and research laboratory, the most important of which are saving of time, money, and space. The chemist who uses microliter methods in his laboratory knows that an analysis can often be performed in one-half of the time required for macroprocedures. Less space is needed for equipment because it can conveniently be placed on the laboratory bench within reach of the technician.

Most microcentrifuges are capable of speeds up to 20,000 rpm with centrifugal forces of about 25,000 g. They accelerate to maximum speed within 15–30 seconds and need little time to stop; this cuts the time for centrifugation to a few minutes. Pipetting of small volumes, especially with constriction pipets, is several times faster than pipetting of ml quantities. An outsider may not understand these considerations, but time saving is a decisive factor considering the workload in a routine laboratory.

Micromethods save chemicals. Modern analytical techniques require expensive biochemicals such as enzymes, substrates and coenzymes; a substantial relief in the budget is felt when only one tenth of the otherwise necessary quantities is consumed. In increasing numbers clinical laboratories introduce microliter procedures into their routine program and several perform microliter methods exclusively.

The accuracy of a microliter method is equal to the accuracy of the macromethod from which it was adapted. The experimental error of methods in the clinical laboratory is usually between 0.5–5%. Experience in our laboratory has shown that, even with ultramicro procedures which include the weighing of tissue samples in mμg-quantities, the coefficient of variation rarely exceeds 5%. The error of the chemical analysis *per se* is not greater than 2–3%.

Thorough training in microliter methods is of course essential. A capable technician can learn microanalysis within three to four weeks.

Only a few technicians and academically trained chemists do not develop the skill for these methods. With the techniques mastered, the results of the analyses will depend mainly on the quality of the technical tools.

Until a few years ago it was left to the chemist to develop his own or to modify existing instruments and tools for microanalysis. The work of the pioneers in this field, H. Holter, O. H. Lowry, D. Glick and P. Kirk (to name a few) was the guidepost for most developments. Industry has now caught up with the many requests for special instrumentation and most of the equipment essential to the microanalytical laboratory is now commercially available.

Chapter 2

Equipment for Microliter Analysis

PHOTOMETERS

Photometric measurements with microcuvettes require a photometer with an adapter to confine the light beam to a cross-section narrow enough to pass through the liquid without touching the walls of the cuvette or the meniscus of the fluid. This is achieved by a simple pinhole or slit diaphragm*, or, to avoid a substantial loss of light, by an optical system.

A number of spectrophotometers and filter photometers with accessories for microliter analysis are commercially available, and their discussion is based on the author's personal experience.

Zeiss spectrophotometer PMQII

A special sample changer for microliter cuvettes with a built-in optical system (Figure 2) is available for this instrument (Figure 1). The optical system permits most of the light issuing from the monochromator to traverse tubular microcells up to a length of 5 cm. The spectral band

* Lowry, O. H., J. Biol. Chem. **163**, 633 (1946).

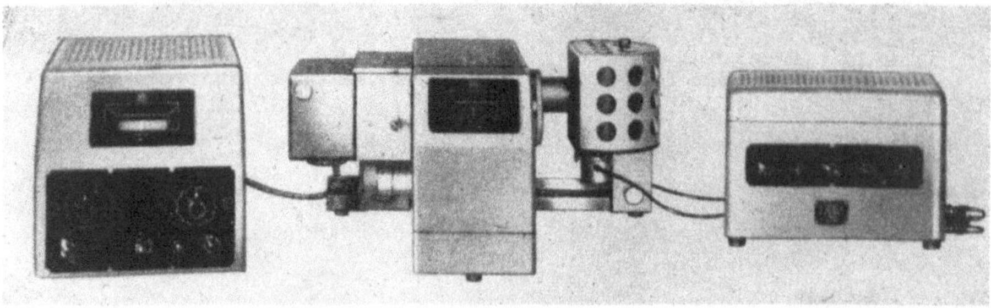

Figure 1. Zeiss Spectrophotometer PMQ II (Carl Zeiss, West Germany, Carl Zeiss, Inc., New York, New York).

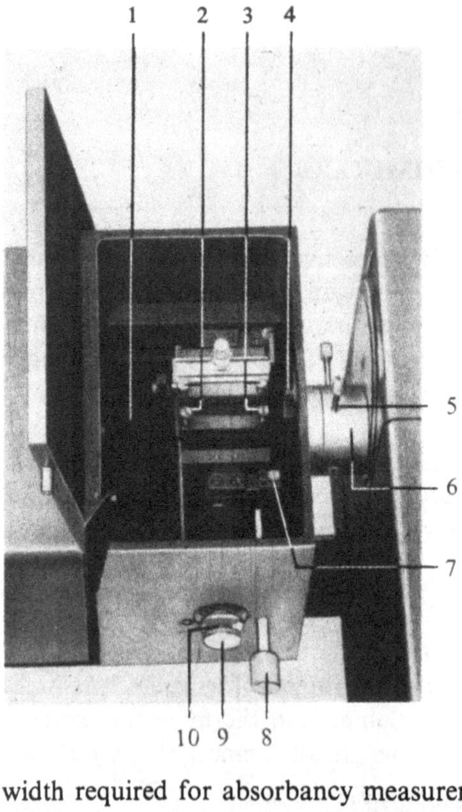

Figure 2. Sample changer for PMQ II with inserted microcuvette

1. short tube for reception of lens
2. and 3. screws for adjusting the height of the cuvette support
4. cross-hole screw for holding and adjusting lens
5. screws for adjusting lens
6. tubular adapter
7. screw for lateral adjustment of the cuvette support
8. pull rod for the cuvette changer
9. knurled screw for limiting the lateral movement of the cuvettes
10. lock nut.

width required for absorbancy measurements with the microcell equipment only needs to be increased by the factor of 1.7, as compared with macrocells and similar amplification. The sample changer can be fitted

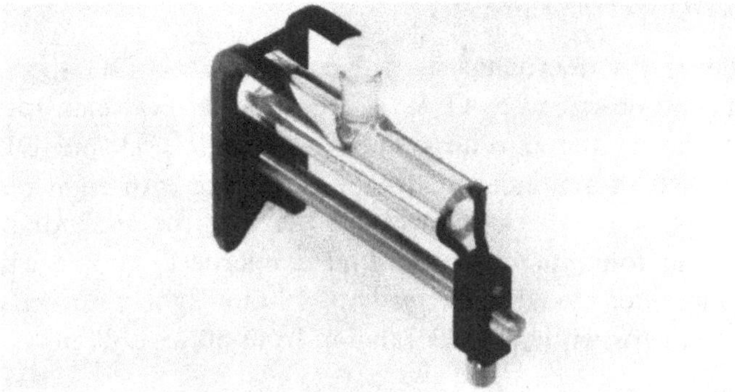

Figure 3a. Tubular microcuvette with holder

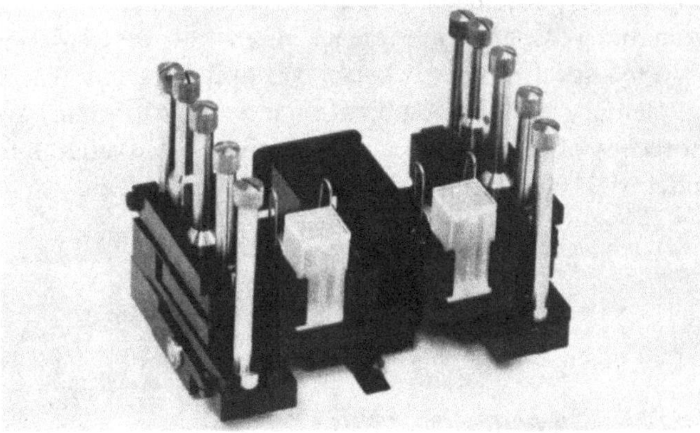

Figure 3b. Trough microcuvette with holder

with holders for trough microcells (Figure 3). Microcells with an inside width of 4 mm and up to 5 cm in length and microcells with 2 mm inside width and up to 1 cm length can be used with the optical system if the monochromator slit is not opened more than 0.8 mm. Precise adjustment of the microliter cells is easy to achieve by a built-in magnetic device. With careful adjustment the amount of sample required is 200 μl/cm light path for the 4-mm and 100 μl/cm light path for the 2-mm microliter cuvette.

In the clinical laboratory, trough-type microliter cuvettes are preferred, mainly because optical enzyme tests, which require mixing of the assay medium in the cuvette, can be performed more easily than in tubular microcells. The standard cuvette changer (without optical system) can be fitted with a movable slit diaphragm having four different slit widths, and a magnetic positioner for independent adjustment of four trough microliter cuvettes.

Beckman DU spectrophotometer

An adapter for microanalysis with the Beckman DU spectrophotometer was first described by O. H. Lowry in 1946. Beckman Instruments now furnishes a microcuvette system for models DU and DU 2. The system consists of a circular micro-aperture plate with eight pinholes of various sizes, a microcell holder with devices for individual vertical adjustment of four microcuvettes, and a microcell sample carrier. Six sizes of microliter trough cuvettes with 10-mm light path are available for measurements with volumes ranging from 50 to 1200 μl.

Eppendorf Photometer

The Eppendorf photometer (Figure 4) is equipped with a series of monochromatic glass and interference filters for the isolation of the commonly used spectral lines between 313 and 1014 nm. The radiation source is a mercury vapor or combination mercury-cadmium vapor lamp. Three photocells of different spectral sensitivity are available for model 1100; model M 1100 is equipped with a photomultiplier.

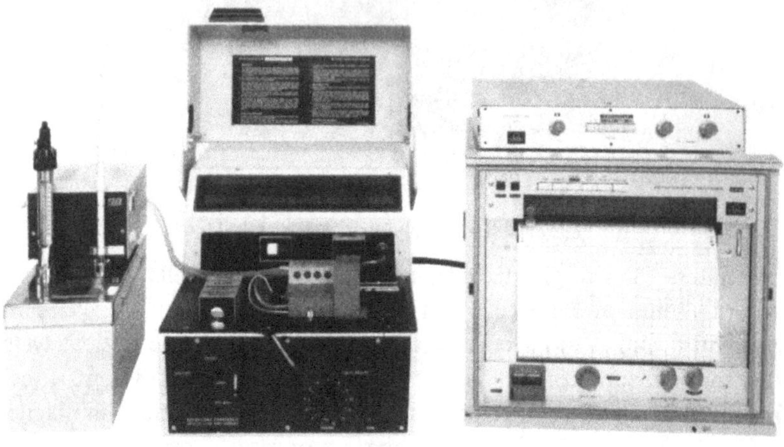

Figure 4. Eppendorf Photometer with recording accessory.
(Netheler & Hinz, Hamburg, West Germany, Brinkmann Instruments, USA).

The cuvette holder receives three cuvettes. A slit diaphragm is supplied for use with microcuvettes of 2-mm width and a light path of 10, 20 and 40 mm. With careful vertical adjustment the minimum volume required in microcells is 110 μl per 10 mm length. The Eppendorf photometer employs direct reading of absorbance with partial compensation by a set of calibrated resistances. The ready accessibility of the cuvettes permits quick operation with this precise, stable and sturdy instrument.

Gilford spectrophotometers

Trough-type microliter cuvettes with 10-mm light paths can be used with the various Gilford spectrophotometer models. Pinhole diaphragms and a special cell holder for independent vertical adjustment of four microliter cells permit the reduction of the working volume to about 40 μl.

The Gilford 300 and 300-N microsample spectrophotometer is designed for speedy operation, and it features an automatic sampling system which permits about five samples to be read per minute. The 10-mm microcuvette holds a volume of only 120 μl, but at least 500 μl sample are needed for filling. This fact unfortunately excludes this instrument for use in the majority of the microliter methods described in this book, most of which have a final assay volume between 200 and 300 μl.

A model 300-N was tested in our laboratory and the performance was as described by the manufacturer. It would seem possible that the manufacturer could redesign the sampling system in order to eliminate some of the dead space and to reduce the required filling volume to 200–250 μl.

Spectronic 20 (Bausch and Lomb)

The Spectronic 20 is equipped with a diffraction grating system and a tungsten lamp as radiation source. The wavelength can be set between 340 and 650 nm, and the range can be extended by use of a filter and a different photo-tube. A special cuvette holder receives a 100-μl cuvette with 10-mm light path.

The instrument tested in the author's laboratory had a slightly unstable zero point. It is therefore suggested that a second cuvette holder with a cuvette filled with water or reagent blank to permit frequent checking and readjusting of the zero point be available. The scale, absorbance, and % transmission is small, and exact reading, particularly of the absorbance, is therefore difficult.

Beckman-Spinco 151 Spectro-colorimeter

This instrument is part of the Beckman-Spinco Ultramicro Analytical System (page 29) designed by Sanz. A glass wedge interference filter covers the wavelength between 400 and 600 nm. The small scale (absorbance and %-transmission) does not permit exact reading. The 100-μl cuvette is stationary and connected to a suction pump for evacuation. The light path of only 6.4 mm is a decisive disadvantage and leads to low and inaccurate reading with many color reactions.

The instrument tested in our laboratory was unstable, and the reproducibility of various microanalyses was unsatisfactory. Reports from other authors are more favorable, however, and we must mention that we probably had a poorly functioning instrument at our disposal.

The basic idea of Sanz for a microphotometer is certainly a good one. One can only hope that the manufacturer revises the construction of this instrument, particularly because other parts of the analytical system are very useful.

SPECIAL DEVICES FOR PHOTOMETRY

Automated photometers

Automatic cuvette changers are available for several photometers. They permit continuous and simultaneous recording of absorbance changes in four to six cuvettes.

Self-emptying microcuvettes

Self-emptying microcuvettes operated in connection with a suction pump are available for some of the photometers. The carry-over from the previous sample normally does not exceed 1% of the volume, and rinsing between samples is unnecessary unless samples with great absorbance differences are measured in succession. In this case prerinsing with about 50 μl of the following sample is suggested. In serial analyses in our laboratory we prefer to empty the cuvettes by suction from the top. The cuvettes are left in the cell holder and the fluid is removed with polyethylene tubing attached to a strong vacuum pump. After the fluid is removed, the cuvette is flushed once with water: by moving the tubing up and down and back and forth several times, the water can be completely removed.

An automatic filling and emptying device is available for the Spectronic 20, but it is not suited for microliter analysis. Although the cuvette holds only 100 μl, 1.5 ml of sample are needed for flushing and filling.

Zeiss microcuvette MR 1 D

This special cuvette holds 20 μl and is designed as a flow-through cell (Figure 5), but a simple device can be made in the laboratory to measure single samples: one of the outlets is fitted with a 2–3-cm long piece of polyethylene tubing. With the technique described on page 17 (constriction pipets), press in a constriction a few millimeters above the outlet, using a pair of pliers shown in Figure 10. To the other outlet fit a longer piece of tubing and attach to it a three-way stopcock. Connect one outlet of the cock to a suction pump, the other to a Hamilton microliter syringe. To fill the cuvette, use a polyethylene pipet with a long tip to transfer between 30 and 35 μl of sample into the tubing with the constriction. With the cuvette in the light beam, draw the fluid slowly

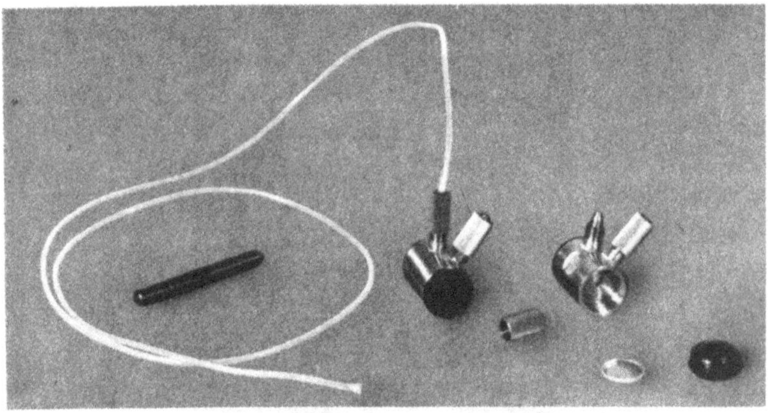

Figure 5. Zeiss microcuvette MR 1D. Volume 20 μl. Designed as a flow-through cuvette; use for single measurements is possible (see text).

into the cuvette with the syringe, and watch the indicator scale. As long as the cuvette is not completely filled or air bubbles trapped, the absorbance will be extremely high. By carefully moving the plunger back and forth, one will find an absorbance minimum when the cuvette is filled completely and bubble-free. The cuvette is flushed and rinsed by suction.

This technique is of course not recommended for routine measurements, but it can be used for special purposes when very little sample is available.

Temperature-controlled cell holders

Enzyme determinations, with the optical test, performed directly in the cuvette, require a temperature-controlled cell holder. These holders or thermospacers are available for most instruments. A special holder is needed for the short microliter cuvette, which we prefer in our laboratory. The temperature-controlled cuvette holder furnished with the Eppendorf photometer can be adapted for the use with microliter cuvettes by taking off the upper half of the two-piece metal block.

MICROCENTRIFUGES

Basically any laboratory centrifuge can be used with micro test tubes by fitting a reducing holder (liner) to the existing centrifuge shields (Figure 6 shows such a holder made from Plexiglas to receive 12 micro

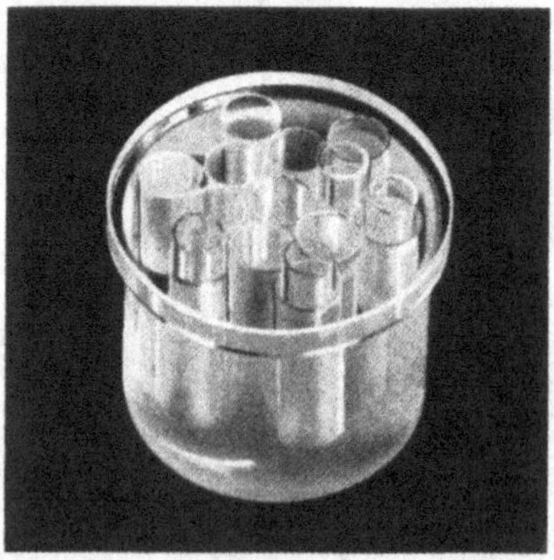

Figure 6. Reducing insert for centrifuging micro test tubes in an ordinary laboratory centrifuge.

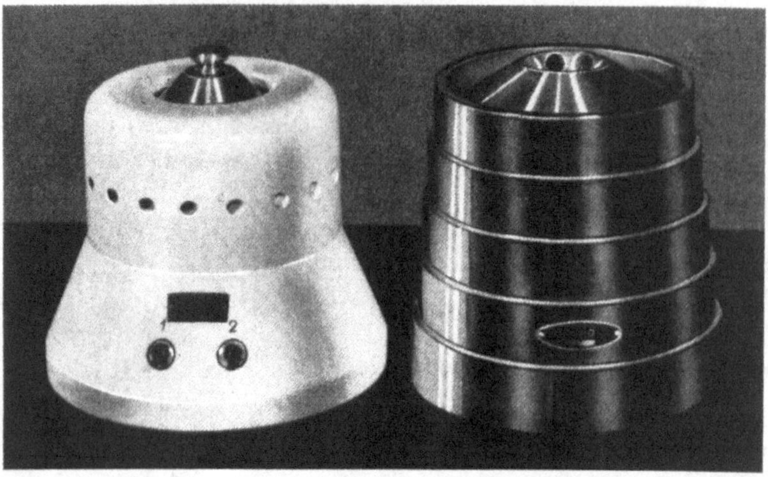

Figure 7. Microcentrifuges
left: Old Dick, Brøndby Strand, Denmark
right: Microchemical Specialties, Berkeley, California.

test tubes). Several useful high-speed microcentrifuges are commercially available. The centrifuges of Misco and O. Dick (Figure 7) are angle-head units which attain forces of up to 22,000 and 15,000 g respectively. The Misco centrifuge accommodates 8 micro test tubes with up to 1 ml capacity, while the O. Dick centrifuge accommodates 12 test tubes with up to 0.5 ml capacity.

Microcentrifuges supplied with the Beckman-Spinco Ultramicro Analytical System (page 29) and the Eppendorf Microliter System (page 30) accommodate the special micro test tubes of the respective system only.

MICROPIPETS

Pipets with volumes from about 1–500 μl are called micropipets or lambda (λ) pipets (1 μl = 1 λ = 0.001 ml). Of the various designs of commercially available micropipets, we prefer and strongly recommend the constriction pipet (Figure 8). This pipet was developed at Carlsberg

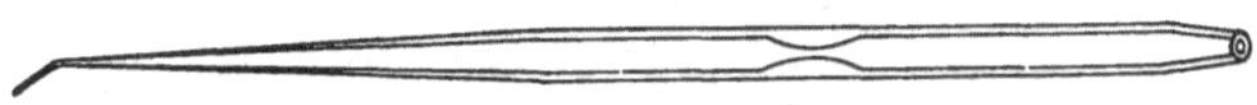

Figure 8. Sketch of a glass constriction pipet.

Laboratory by Levy[1] (Carlsberg pipet) and first described as being made from glass. The pipets are operated by mouth with a rubber tube. The inside diameter of the pipet tip and the inside diameter of the constriction must be well-balanced to assure that the meniscus of the fluid assumes a reproducible position at the constriction. With the pipet in a vertical position, gravity should force fluid drawn above the constriction to drop down to it but not farther. For delivery a slight pressure is applied. Pipets with volumes of 1 μl and larger are on the market; smaller pipets must be specifically ordered or made in the laboratory. Commercial constriction pipets vary in quality especially in regard to the tips.[2]

The mean standard deviation of the volumes delivered from glass constriction pipets increases as expected with decreasing pipet volumes (page 38).

Two types of micropipets made from polyethylene were developed in

[1] Levy, M., Z. Physiol. Chem. **240**, 33 (1936). The pipets are also known as Lang-Levy pipets.

[2] Lang-Levy type pipets are available from many instrument supply houses.

our laboratory: (a) capillary pipets[1] with volumes from 0.1 μl to 5 μl and (b) constriction pipets[2] with volumes from < 1 μl to about 300 μl. Polyethylene pipets have several advantages over glass pipets: the accuracy of delivery of fluid is increased because polyethylene is hydrophobic; they can be made with ease; they are unbreakable. Polyethylene has a melting point of about 115°C and can best be molded at temperatures between 40–70°C.

Capillary pipets

This type of pipet consists of a polyethylene capillary mounted in a glass tube support. The supports are 8–10 cm long with an inside diameter of about 1.8 mm and an outside diameter of about 3 mm. Polyethylene tubing with 0.5 mm inside and about 1 mm outside diameter is best suited for pipets from 1 μl to 5 μl.

To draw a very fine tip having an inside diameter of about 0.1 mm, the tubing is heated and slowly rotated over a small flame. As soon as the material becomes soft, the tubing is pulled gently with tension maintained until the polyethylene cools. The tip is then cut to a length of a few millimeters. From the inside diameter of the tubing and the desired volume, the necessary length is approximately calculated; the tubing is cut accordingly at the free end with a razor blade, allowing a few millimeters in excess. The pipet is then mounted in the support and the volume determined colorimetrically (page 36). The volume can be adjusted by cutting off thin sections from the rear of the tubing.

The glass tube supports are prepared in the following way. One end is allowed to collapse in a hot flame, producing an opening just wide enough to receive the polyethylene pipet. In the upper third of the tube a constriction of 5–10 mm in length is made by heating and rotating the glass over a hot flame. The constriction must be narrow enough to insure slow filling and emptying of the pipet. With the tip of the polyethylene pipet immersed in water, air should bubble slowly when light pressure is applied with a mouth tube. The ready-made pipet is shown in Figure 9. The polyethylene pipet is mounted to extend about 2–3 mm free into the support. In addition to the straight pipet a slightly bent model is used. The outside diameter of the support is such that fluid from the pipet can be delivered on the wall in the lower part of 4.5 × 30-mm micro test tubes. For pipets with volumes smaller than 1 μ, capillaries with an inside diameter of 0.1–0.2 mm are drawn from

[1] Mattenheimer, H., and K. Borner, Mikrochim. Acta **1959**, 917.
[2] Mattenheimer, H., J. Lab. Clin. Med. **58**, 783 (1961).

wider polyethylene tubing. The pipets are operated with mouth tubing. Because of the capillary attraction, complete and reproducible filling is easy. Fluid is delivered quantitatively.

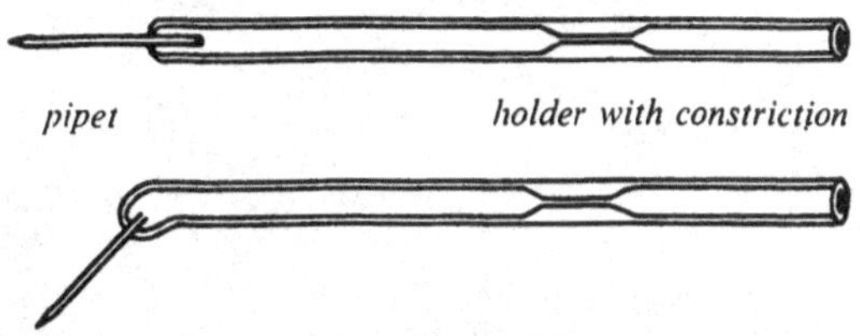

Figure 9. Polyethylene capillary pipet with glass holder.

Constriction pipets

Selection of polyethylene tubing

pipet volume (μl)	diameter (mm) outside	inside
0.5–2	1	0.6
1–10	1.3	0.8
10–50	2.8	1.6
50 a. over	3.4	2.1

Pulling the tip

A piece of tubing is rotated while being heated approximately 3 cm from one end high over a small flame. As soon as the material becomes soft, the tubing is pulled carefully at one or both ends and tension is maintained until the polyethylene is cool. The tip can then be cut to the desired length.

Pressing the constriction

For pipets with volumes $< 10\ \mu l$, a simple cable stripper with carefully polished edges is used to press the constriction (Figure 10). For pipets with volumes $> 10\ \mu l$, a pair of forming pliers was developed* (Figure 11). The desired volume of water is aspirated into the pipet either from a balance pan or directly from a calibrated pipet. The position at which the constriction will be made is marked with a grease pencil 1 or 2 mm above the water meniscus. The pipet is then emptied and dried. The

* The forming pliers may be obtained from ACME Model Works, Inc., 200 N. Jefferson Street, Chicago, Illinois.

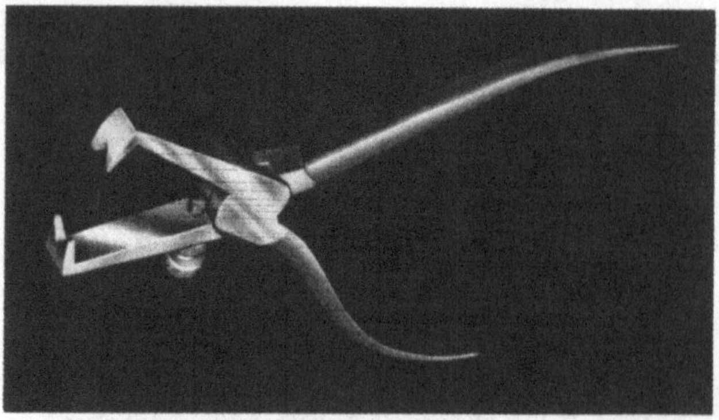

Figure 10. Cable stripping pliers with ground edges used for forming the constriction in polyethylene pipets < 10 μl. When closed the jaws overlap.

pliers are heated in boiling water, and the constriction is pressed in at the marked point. The pliers are kept closed for about 2 minutes and are then cooled under running tap water before being opened. One point is of critical importance. On each side of the constriction a "wing" is

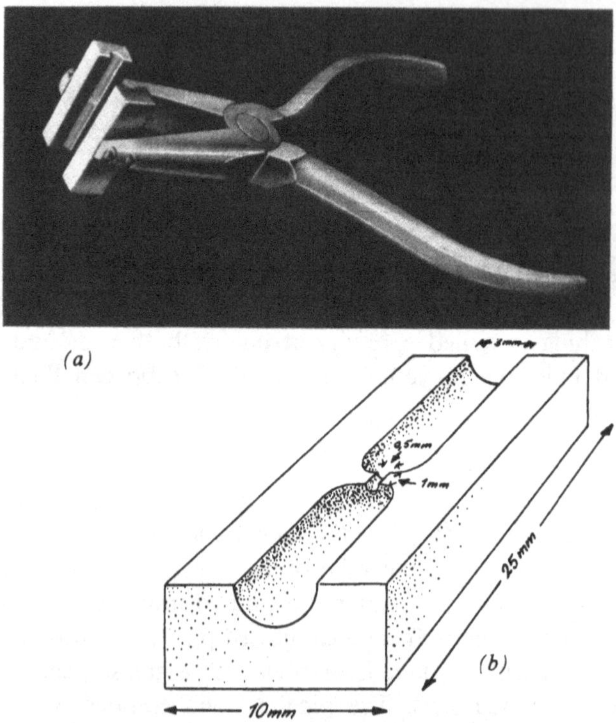

Figure 11. (a) Pair of forming pliers for pipets > 10 μl. (b) Sketch of one of the two identical mold halves.

formed, consisting of two laminae (Figure 12). Unless these have been firmly bonded after heating, fluid will be sucked between the laminae. The constriction should be checked under the microscope and the pipets discarded if the laminae are open. If the constriction has been made properly, the fluid meniscus will be held at the narrowest point of constriction, except when an increase of pressure is applied to overcome the resistance. The pipets are operated by mouth, using rubber tubing. The ends of very thin pipets must be inserted in polyethylene tubing with a wider bore and wider outside diameter, to which the rubber tubing can be fitted for suction. Polyethylene tubing from various suppliers varies in quality. Some brands have to be rinsed with a detergent before the constriction is pressed in.

We have used polyethylene constriction pipets in our laboratory for

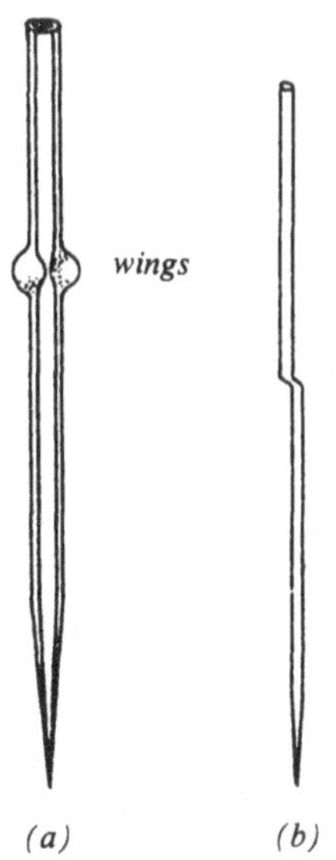

Figure 12. Polyethylene constriction pipets
(a) Model for volumes > 10 μl. The "wings" are formed when the constriotion is pressed in with a pair of molding pliers (Figure 11) and consist of two laminae which have to be joined in a firm bond (see text).
(b) Model for volumes < 10 μl. The steplike constriction is formed with the pliers shown in Figure 10.

over eight years. The pipets do not change their volume over a period of time, some of the first ones we made are still in use. Because heat widens the constriction, polyethylene pipets must not be rinsed with hot water and must not be used to pipet hot solutions.

Calibration of the pipets

Pipets with volumes > 10 μl can be calibrated gravimetrically with water; smaller pipets are calibrated colorimetrically with *p*-nitrophenol in alkaline solution (page 36). Corrections for too large a volume can be made by cutting a piece from the tip. Otherwise the pipets are used with a correction factor. With practice the desired volume can be attained within ± 2 or 3 per cent.

Sanz pipets

The overflow pipet designed by Sanz is part of the Beckman-Spinco Analytical System (page 29). The pipet is a piece of polyethylene tubing, with a tip at one end and mounted in a glass dome screwed onto a polyethylene bottle. Pipets of various sizes, ranging from 0.5–250 μl, are available. Because polyethylene is hydrophobic, the menisci of the fluid are easy to adjust at both ends of the pipet. Operation is simple. Type A (Figure 13) is used to pipet the sample. The bottle is squeezed gently and the opening in the dome is then closed with the forefinger. The sample is aspirated by very slowly releasing the pressure until a small drop flows over. At that moment the forefinger is removed from the hole and the pressure slowly released. To deliver, the hole is closed and the bottle squeezed gently. With pipets made from a high quality polyethylene

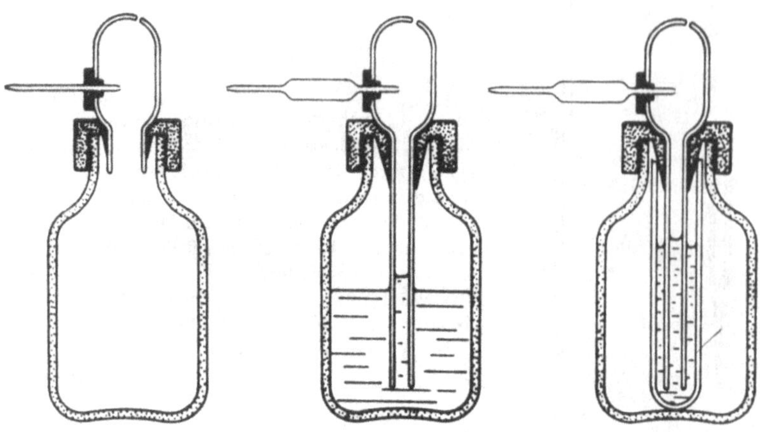

A B C

Figure 13. SANZ-pipets. *A*: sample pipet, *B* and *C*: reagent pipets.

(see above), no droplets will remain in the pipet. Some pipets included in reagent kits (Chempak) which we purchased from Beckman-Spinco could in our experience not be completely emptied. After replacing the tubing with a different brand of polyethylene, the pipets worked to satisfaction. According to Sanz [Chemica **13**, 192 (1959)], it is not necessary to rinse the sample pipet between samples because droplets that may remain are flushed out with the overflowing drop of the next sample. We recommend rinsing once with redistilled water. For cleaning the pipets, see page 33.

Two types of reagent pipets are shown in Figure 13. For solutions which cannot be stored in polyethylene bottles, a test tube is inserted into the bottle (C). Reagent is pipetted by closing the hole in the dome with the forefinger and squeezing the bottle until the fluid has filled the pipet and the first drop flows over. The hole is then opened and the pressure released; the overflow is wiped off. The fluid is delivered from the pipet by closing the hole and squeezing the bottle gently. Although operating the pipet is simple, working over a long period of time may lead to weariness of the hand and inaccurate pipetting.

Eppendorf microliter pipet

The Eppendorf microliter pipet is a piston pipet available in eight models dispensing fixed volumes (5, 10, 20, 50, 100, 200, 500, and 1000 μl). The exchangeable tips are made from polypropylene. The spring-loaded piston is activated by a push-button control which is easily manipulated by the thumb (Figure 14). The operating technique is described in Figure 15. According to the manufacturer, the coefficient of variation for pipets of 50–1000 μl is less than 0.3% and increases to about 0.8% for the 5-μl pipets. With our pipets we found a slightly higher coefficient for the 5- and 10-μl pipet. The Eppendorf microliter pipet can be highly recommended for routine analysis, and it is part of the Eppendorf Microliter System (page 30).

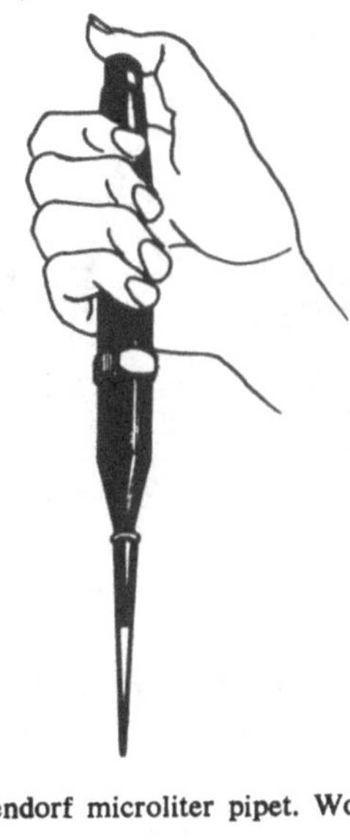

Figure 14. Eppendorf microliter pipet. Working position.

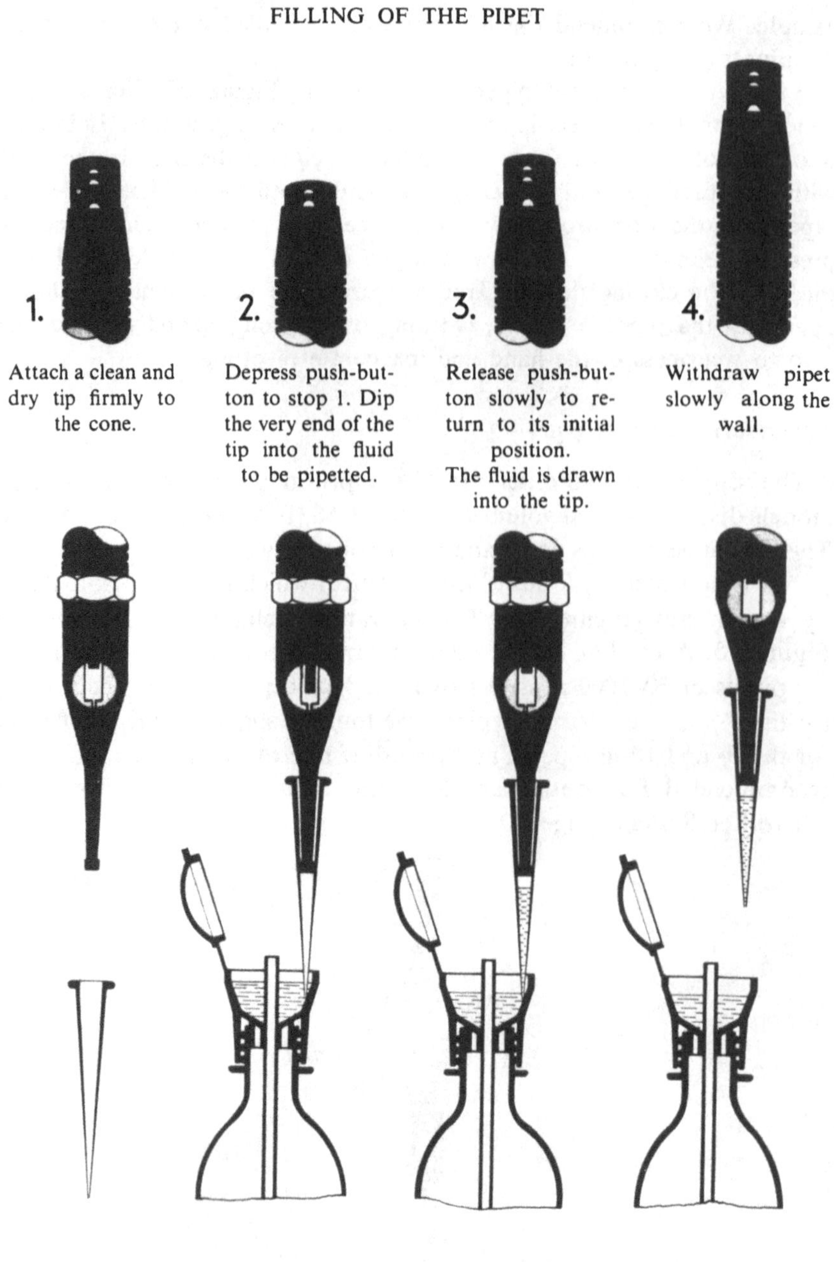

Figure 15. Eppendorf microliter pipet. Operating technique.

DISPENSING

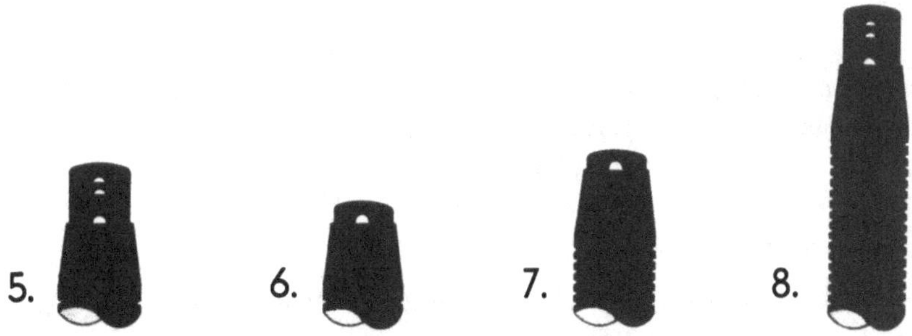

5. Place tip on the wall of the test tube.

6. Depress push-button to stop 1, wait at least one second and depress to stop 2.

7. With the push-button still at stop 2 withdraw pipet slowly along the wall.

8. Release push-button to return to its initial position.

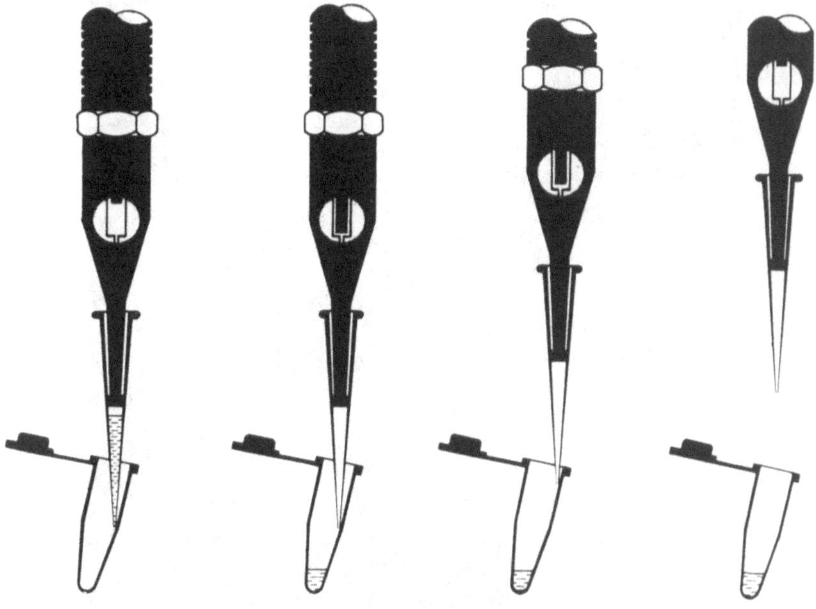

MIXING AND STIRRING DEVICES

Mixing of small volumes is critical. If one adds, *e.g.*, 5 μl of a dye solution to 50 μl water in a micro test tube, homogeneous mixing can hardly be achieved without some kind of mixing device. The following devices can be recommended.

Magnetic stirrers

Glass spherules filled with iron powder ("fleas") and operated by a strong magnet are well suited for mixing and stirring in micro test tubes (Figure 16).

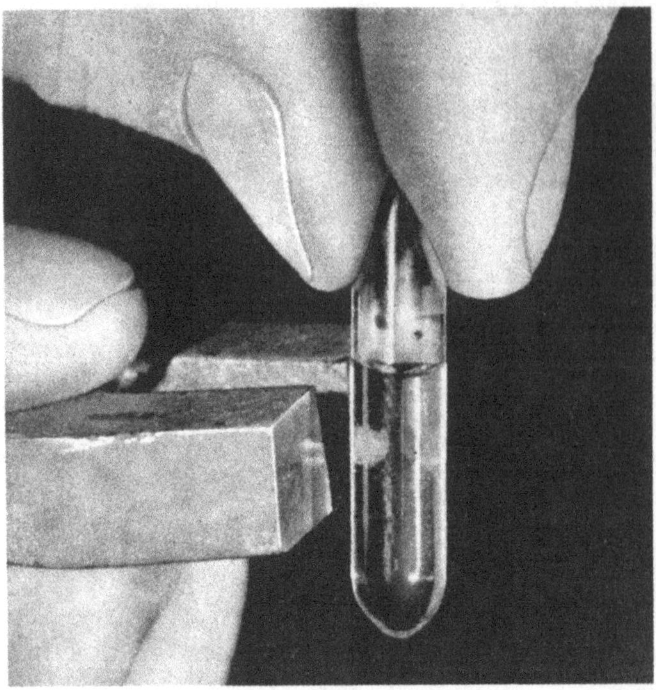

Figure 16. Mixing with a magnetic stirrer (flea). The flea is moved up and down with a strong magnet. In silicone-coated tubes separated droplets can be quantitatively collected by the flea.

Figure 17 shows the steps involved in making the "fleas." Glass capillaries (Ø outside *ca.* 1.2 mm, Ø inside *ca.* 1 mm) are fused in a flame at one end (1). The closed end is then carefully heated by holding the tip close to the flame of a microburner. Light pressure is applied from a mouth tube in order to blow a bubble of about 2 mm in diameter (2). The spherule is filled with iron dust to just over one-half. Powder remaining in the capillary is brought down into the spherule with the aid of a magnet (3). The capillary is attached to a vacuum pump and melted off with the vacuum applied (4). The flea is then melted off with a small pointed flame. The remaining pedicle should be as short as possible (5). Spontaneous bursting by expansion is avoided because the spherule is under vacuum.

The fleas are cleaned as described on page 34. Fleas with a crack absorb water during washing; these rust and then must be discarded.

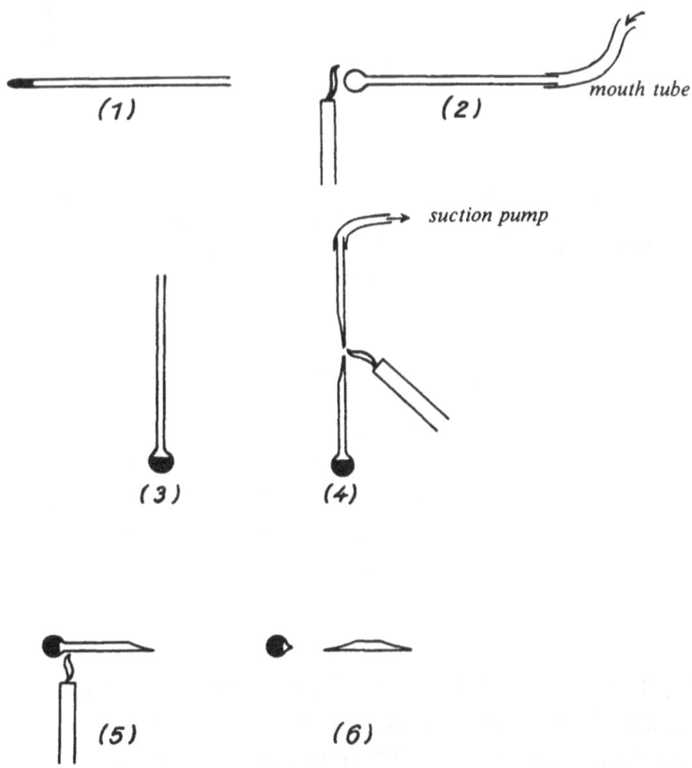

Figure 17. Procedure to produce magnetic stirrers (fleas). Explanation: see text.

Fleas may also be made from a piece of iron wire (*e.g.*, paper clip) and polyethylene tubing. Approximately 1-mm long pieces of wire are cut and inserted into pieces of thin polyethylene tubing about 3 mm long. The protruding ends of the tubing are welded by clamping with a hot pair of tweezers. The fleas are left in water overnight; those with a leak absorb water and corrode.

A device for simultaneous stirring of several micro test tubes is shown in Figure 18.

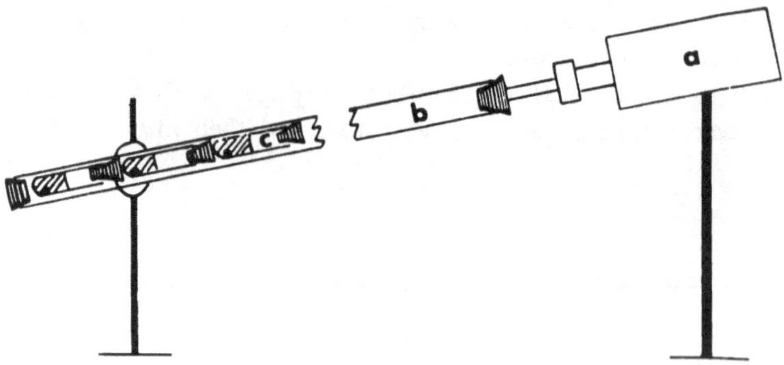

Figure 18. Device for simultaneous mixing in several micro test tubes. (a) Adjustable electric motor; (b) Glass tubing to receive the micro test tubes; (c) Micro test tubes filled not more than one-half, closed with rubber stoppers; each tube contains a flea or a glass bead.

Polyethylene stirring rods

To avoid scratching of the cuvette windows, polyethylene stirring rods are used instead of glass stirrers for mixing in microcuvettes. The ends of 4–6-cm long pieces of thin polyethylene tubing are welded by clamping with a hot pair of tweezers. A piece of wire may be inserted to stiffen the stirrer.

Vibrators

A simple vibrator, consisting of a high-speed electric motor to which is attached a slightly eccentric metal cone is shown in Figure 19. Micro test tubes which may not be filled more than half are held between two fingers; their upper third is pressed firmly against the rotating rod. Various vibrators with eccentric rubber heads are commercially available. Special vibrators were developed for the Beckman-Spinco Ultramicro Analytical System (page 29) and the Eppendorf Microliter System (page 31).

Two methods described in this book (see pages 185 and 210) require a simple massage vibrator for mixing. The massage head is removed and replaced by a holder for micro test tubes. The vibration must be controlled by a powerstat to avoid splashing of the liquid in the micro test tube.

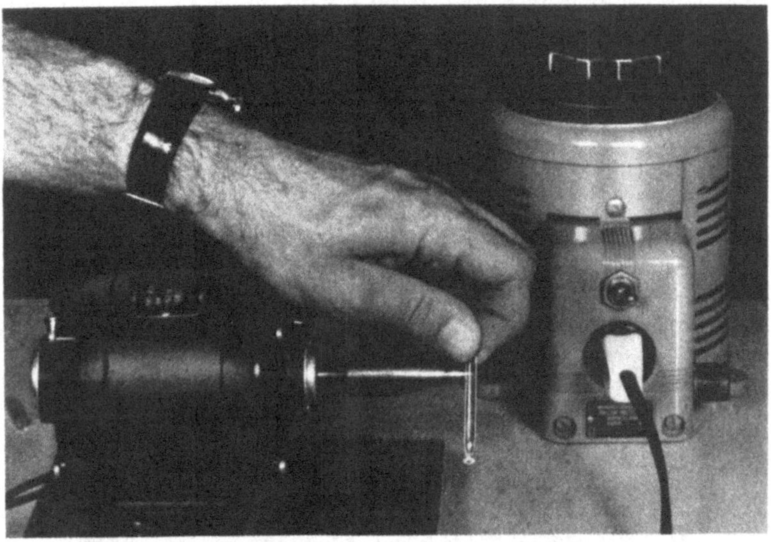

Figure 19. "Buzzer" vibrator for mixing in micro test tubes. Details: see text.

MICROBURETS

For microtitration methods described in this book, a microburet with an accuracy of 0.05–0.1 μl is required. A number of good instruments are on the market. In our laboratory we use and highly recommend the Beckman 153 microtitrator.

MICRO TEST TUBES

The following sizes of micro test tubes, made from Pyrex glass, are suggested for the methods described in this book.

Length (mm)	Inside Diameter (mm)
50	3
30	4.5
50	4.5
50	6.0

The 3 × 50-mm tubes are required for ultramicro procedures (Chapter 8) and should have tapered bottoms. Micro test tubes from polyethylene are manufactured by Beckman-Spinco (400 μl volume) and by Netheler & Hinz (1.5 ml volume).* The latter are available through Brinkmann Instruments.

TEST TUBE RACKS

Micro test tube racks are available from many supply houses. Special racks are part of the Beckman-Spinco Ultramicro Analytical System and the Eppendorf Microliter System.* A rack to hold test tubes and reagent bottles made in the laboratory from Plexiglas is shown in Figure 20.

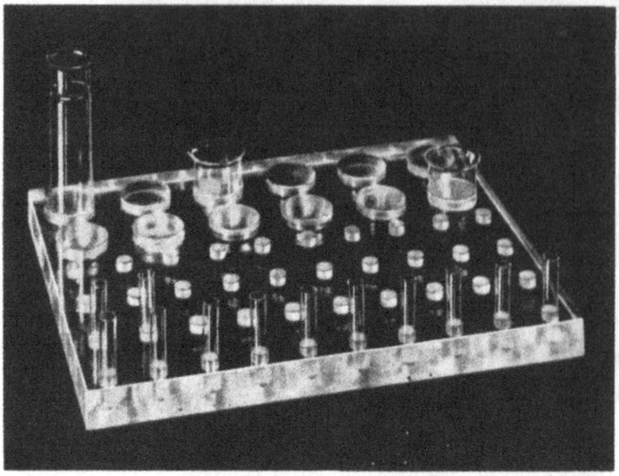

Figure 20. Plexiglas rack for micro test tubes and reagent bottles

MICROANALYTICAL SYSTEMS

Instruments for microanalysis have been combined into sets by several manufacturers. The Beckman-Spinco Ultramicro Analytical System and the Eppendorf Microliter System* were tested in our laboratory.

* Netheler & Hinz, Hamburg, Germany, and Brinkmann Instruments, Westbury, New York.

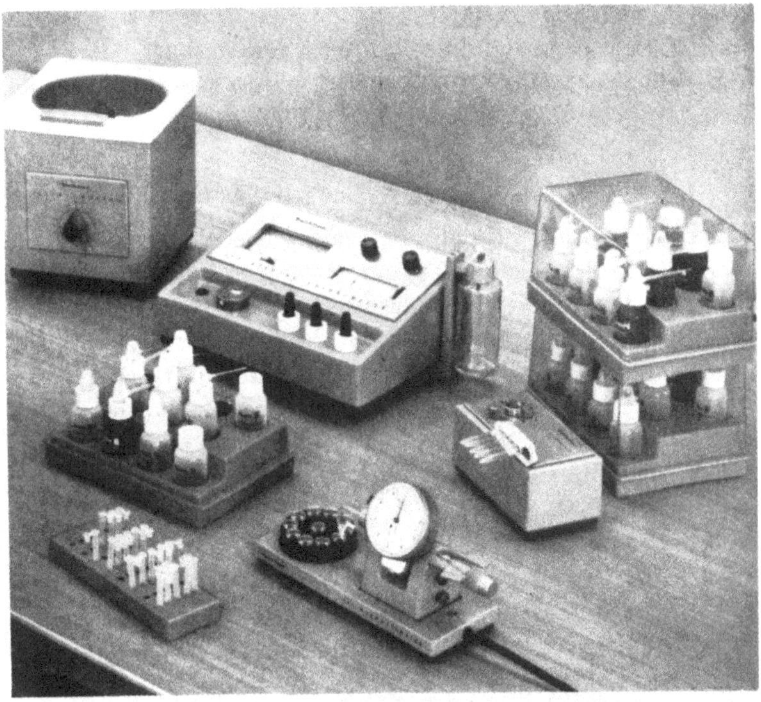

Figure 21. Beckman-Spinco Ultramicro Analytical System.

Beckman-Spinco Ultramicro Analytical System

This system was developed by Sanz. According to the definitions put forward in Chapter 1, it serves for "micro" rather than for "ultramicro" analysis. The system (Figure 21) consists of: spectrocolorimeter, microtitrator, micromixer, microcentrifuge, micropipets, and disposable polyethylene micro test tubes with attached cover.

The system can be recommended except for the spectrocolorimeter, which has certain disadvantages discussed on page 11. Any other photometer suitable for microliter analysis can be used with the system. The microcentrifuge and the Sanz micropipet were discussed on pages 14 and 20, respectively.

The microtitrator is a precision-built instrument with a built-in stirrer; it permits speedy and very accurate titrations. Chloride, for example, can be determined in about 1 minute, including charging of microtitration vessels. The dial can be read accurately to 0.01 μl. We also use this instrument for titrations in micro test tubes, for example, in the glutaminase assay (page 185) to titrate ammonia after microdiffusion.

The micromixer is a vibrator which can be loaded with five Spinco micro test tubes. Mixing in single tubes and tubes of other sizes is achieved by touching the side of the tube with the vibrating bar.

The polyethylene test tubes hold 400 μl, but to achieve proper mixing they should not be filled with more than 300 μl.

Eppendorf Microliter System*

The system consists of (Figure 22): microcuvettes and diaphragm for the Eppendorf photometer, Eppendorf photometer, microcentrifuge, rotary shaker, thermostat, plastic transfer racks for 24 test tubes, Eppendorf micropipets, polyethylene reagent flasks, and disposable solvent- and heat-resistant (up to 120°C) plastic test tubes with attached cover.

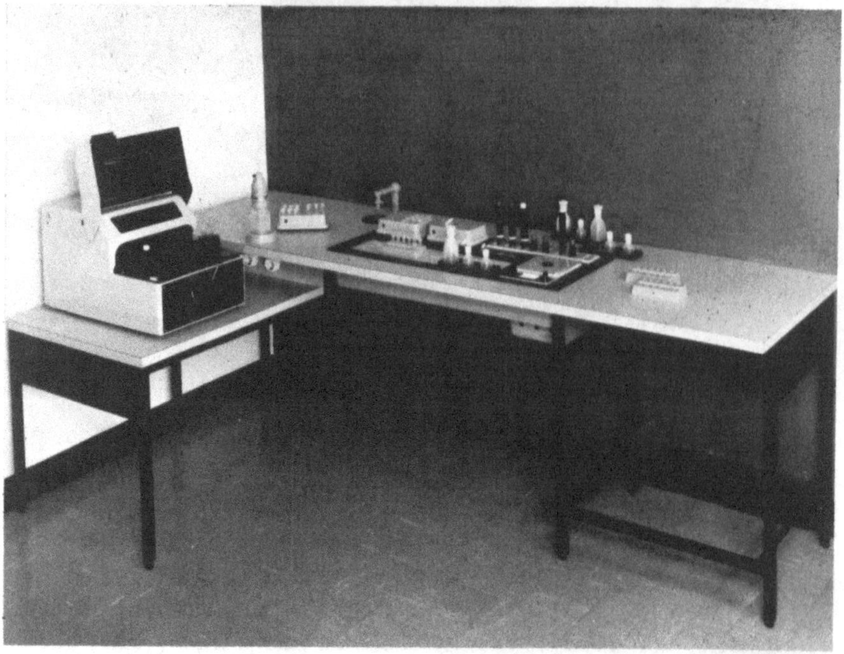

Figure 22. Eppendorf Microliter System.

The Eppendorf photometer with microcuvettes and the micropipets was discussed on pages 10 and 21, respectively. The special test tubes hold 1.5 ml and are wide and short; they are used for all operations, including separation of serum. The plastic transfer rack holds the tubes during filling and all other operations and is used to transport and place the tubes simultaneously on the shaker or the thermostat.

* Netheler & Hinz, Hamburg, Germany, and Brinkmann Instruments, Westbury, New York.

The rotary shaker ensures homogenous mixing within 15–30 seconds. The microcentrifuge can hold 12 tubes and spins at 16,000 rpm (15,000 g). A built-in timer with a setting up to 2 minutes stops the centrifuge automatically. The thermostat operates at 25°, 37°, 56°, and 95°C; tap water can be circulated through a built-in cooling coil. The components of the microliter system, except the photometer, are available mounted in a single desk-top unit which may be built into any existing laboratory bench, or into a special desk-type console with a side table for the photometer. Such a unit permits efficient operation within minimum space.

Chapter 3

General Working Instructions

CLEANING OF GLASSWARE

Glassware is treated with hot half-concentrated HNO_3 and rinsed once with distilled and then with redistilled water. Chromosulfuric acid should be avoided with glassware used for enzyme work. Detergents may be used, but the glassware must be rinsed with acid to remove the thin film which detergents form on the glass surface. Many detergents are enzyme poisons.

Micro test tubes are filled with acid* by packing them into Pyrex glass beaker which fits the shield of a centrifuge. The tubes are covered with acid and filled by centrifuging at not more than 500 rpm. The beaker is then placed in a boiling water bath for 30–60 minutes. The acid is decanted and the tubes are transferred, bottom up, into a beaker fitted with a stainless steel screen supported by a Plexiglas ring (Figure 23). The acid is centrifuged out and drawn from under the screen with suction through a long stainless steel needle. The procedure is repeated four to five times with distilled water and once with redistilled water, heat-

* Lowry, O. H., N. R. Roberts, K. Y. Leiner, M. L. Wu, and A. L. Farr, J. Biol. Chem. **207**, 1 (1954).

ing the tubes filled with water during the second rinse. The tubes are then dried in an oven. Polyethylene pipets are cleaned with detergent. To remove dried residues of blood or serum, soak the pipets in a 5% solution of Na_3PO_4 or in a solution of pepsin in 0.1N HCl. Water is aspirated through to rinse and acetone to dry the pipets. *Warning:* Do not use hot solutions for polyethylene pipets. Glass pipets are treated in the same manner but acid is aspirated through to remove the detergent film.

Magnetic stirrers or fleas made from glass are soaked for one to two hours in *cold* acid. They are then transferred to a fritted disc funnel, washed under suction with plenty of distilled water followed by redistilled water, and rinsed with acetone. The funnel is covered with filter paper and the fleas are dried in the air stream. Polyethylene fleas are soaked in detergent.

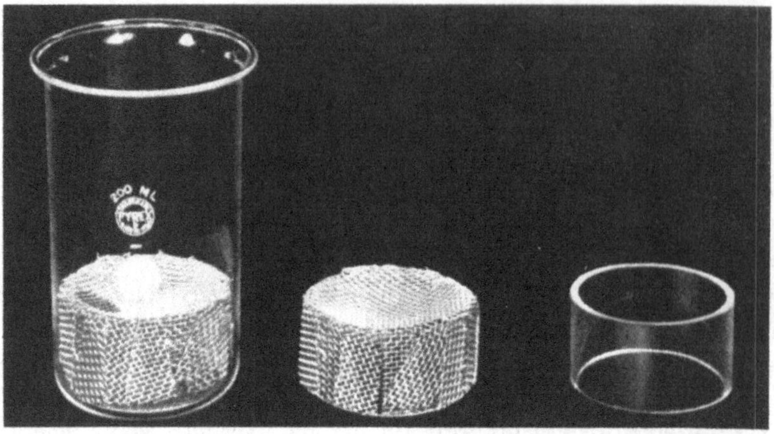

Figure 23. Glass beaker with insert of stainless steel screen for rinsing micro test tubes. The screen is supported by a Plexiglas ring.

SILICONE COATING OF MICRO TEST TUBES

Some methods require micro test tubes with a hydrophobic inner surface to avoid spreading of aqueous fluids. This coating is best done with silicone solutions or silicone pastes. Clean micro test tubes are filled with silicone solution, drained, rinsed with redistilled water, and heated at about 150°C for several hours. Silicone paste is applied with cotton swabs. Excess paste is removed with a dry swab and the tubes are heated at about 150°C. The silicone film should be removed from dirty tubes with toluene prior to cleaning.

FILLING OF MICRO TEST TUBES

After some experience with micromethods, one will learn that working with constriction pipets and micro test tubes is considerably faster and generally more accurate than working with macroequipment. Some critical points need to be mentioned, however. Micropipets are calibrated for blow-out. Gentle blowing is essential to avoid splashing of the fluid. The tip of the pipet must touch the test tube wall (Figure 24a) and be slowly withdrawn along the wall while the fluid is being delivered. When several solutions are pipetted in succession, the tip of the pipet is placed on the wall just above the fluid already delivered, thus making the drops flow together (Figure 24b). To avoid the formation of air bubbles when larger volumes of fluid are delivered into a micro test tube, the tip is

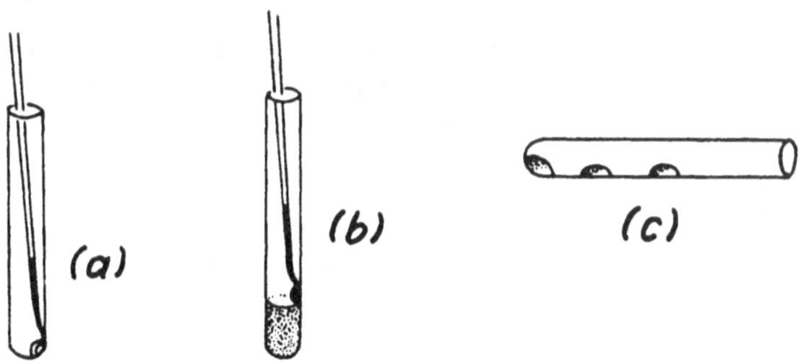

Figure 24. Filling of micro test tubes. Explanations: see text.

placed on the wall close to the bottom, withdrawn slowly and always kept slightly above the fluid surface.

Mixing is achieved by vibration or with a magnetic flea. Droplets that were separated during filling or mixing are recombined with the fluid by short centrifuging at high speed.

Some enzyme methods call for micro test tubes with a hydrophobic inner coating (page 34) in order to keep the buffer, substrate and enzyme solutions separated from each other. The test tube is held horizontally and the solutions are placed on the wall as separate drops (Figure 24c). The drops can be mixed with a magnetic flea or by vibration. This technique has the following advantages:

1. In serial analyses all test tubes are first charged and then mixed simultaneously just prior to incubation.
2. Separate blanks can be prepared by using a magnetic flea to mix buffer and substrate only in one test tube and enzyme and buffer only in another test tube. The tubes are incubated in a horizontal

position to prevent the remaining drop from flowing down. The drop is mixed in just before the reagent to stop the reaction is added.

Micro test tubes are best sealed with parafilm or stoppered with rubber tubing, one end of which is plugged with a glass bead or with a piece of glass tubing sealed at the lower end. To identify the micro test tubes in serial analyses, numbers may be written on the rubber tubing or on small paper strips inserted into the glass tubing used to plug the stopper.

CALIBRATION OF MICROPIPETS

Literature: Borner, K. and H. Mattenheimer, Mikrochim. Acta **1959**, 917; Lowry, O. H., N. R. Roberts, K. Y. Wu, and L. Farr, J. Biol. Chem. **207**,1 (1954).

Micropipets of > 10 μl volume may be calibrated gravimetrically with H_2O, or colorimetrically. Colorimetric calibration with *p*-nitrophenol is recommended for smaller pipets.

Calibration with *p*-nitrophenol

p-Nitrophenol solution, 10.0 mM: in a 100-ml volumetric flask dissolve 139.11 mg recrystallized *p*-nitrophenol with gentle heating in 0.1N NaOH and fill up to the mark.

Standard dilution 1:500: prepare an exact 1:500 dilution of *p*-nitrophenol solution with 0.1N NaOH; use a calibrated pipet and a calibrated volumetric flask.

To calibrate a micropipet, the dilution of the pipet volume with NaOH should be between 1:250 and 1:500.

Example:

The micropipet to be calibrated has a volume of approximately 10 μl. Into at least five test tubes, pipet 5 ml (calibrated pipet) 0.1N NaOH. With the micropipet to be calibrated remove the pipet volume and replace it with 10.0 mM *p*-nitrophenol solution. Read the absorbance of the unknown and of the standard 1:500 dilution in 10-mm cuvettes at 400 nm or a nearby wave-length against 0.1N NaOH as blank.

Calculation:

$$\text{Volume of pipet } (\mu l) = \frac{A_u}{A_{st,\,dil.}} \times DF \times TV$$

where A_u = absorbance of the unknown; $A_{st.\,dil.}$ = absorbance of the standard dilution; DF = dilution factor of the standard dilution (1:500

in example); TV = total volume of the unknown in μl (5000 μl in the example).
In the example: $A_{st.\ dil.} = 0.376$

$A_{400\ nm}^{10\ mm}$	pipet volume
0.376	10.00
0.378	10.05
0.378	10.05
0.381	10.13
0.380	10.10
mean	10.06 μl

Standard deviation: $s = \sqrt{\frac{\Sigma(\bar{x} - x)^2}{n - 1}} = \pm 0.05\ \mu l = \pm 0.49\%$

Standard error of the mean: $s_{\bar{x}} = \sqrt{\frac{\Sigma(\bar{x} - x)^2}{n(n - 1)}} = \pm 0.023\ \mu l = \pm 0.22\%$

The calibration can also be based on the molar extinction coefficient of *p*-nitrophenol $\varepsilon = 18.8 \times 10^3$ 1/mole × cm at 400 nm in alkaline solution. The measurement must then be made at 400 nm and the *p*-nitrophenol solution must be standardized:

$$\frac{A}{\varepsilon \times d} \times 10^3 \times \frac{a}{b} = p\text{-nitrophenol mM}$$

where d = light path in cm
a = total volume of the standard dilution
b = volume of *p*-nitrophenol solution in the standard dilution
x′ = concentration of *p*-nitrophenol solution.

With the suggested 1:500 dilution and 1 cm light path:

$$\frac{A_{st.\ dil.}}{18.8 \times 10^3} \times 10^3 \times \frac{500}{1} = x'\ \text{mM}$$

In the example we find that $A_{st.\ dil.} = 0.376$; $x' = 10.0$ mM.
Calculation for the calibration of microliter pipets:

$$\text{volume of pipet } (\mu l) = \frac{A_u}{18.8} \times \frac{TV\ (\mu l)}{x'}$$

where TV is the total volume of the unknown dilution. Figure 25 shows the standard deviation (s) and the standard error of the mean ($s_{\bar{x}}$) for a number of our pipets. It is evident that the mean error of glass constriction pipets increases considerably more with decreasing volume than the mean error of polyethylene pipets.

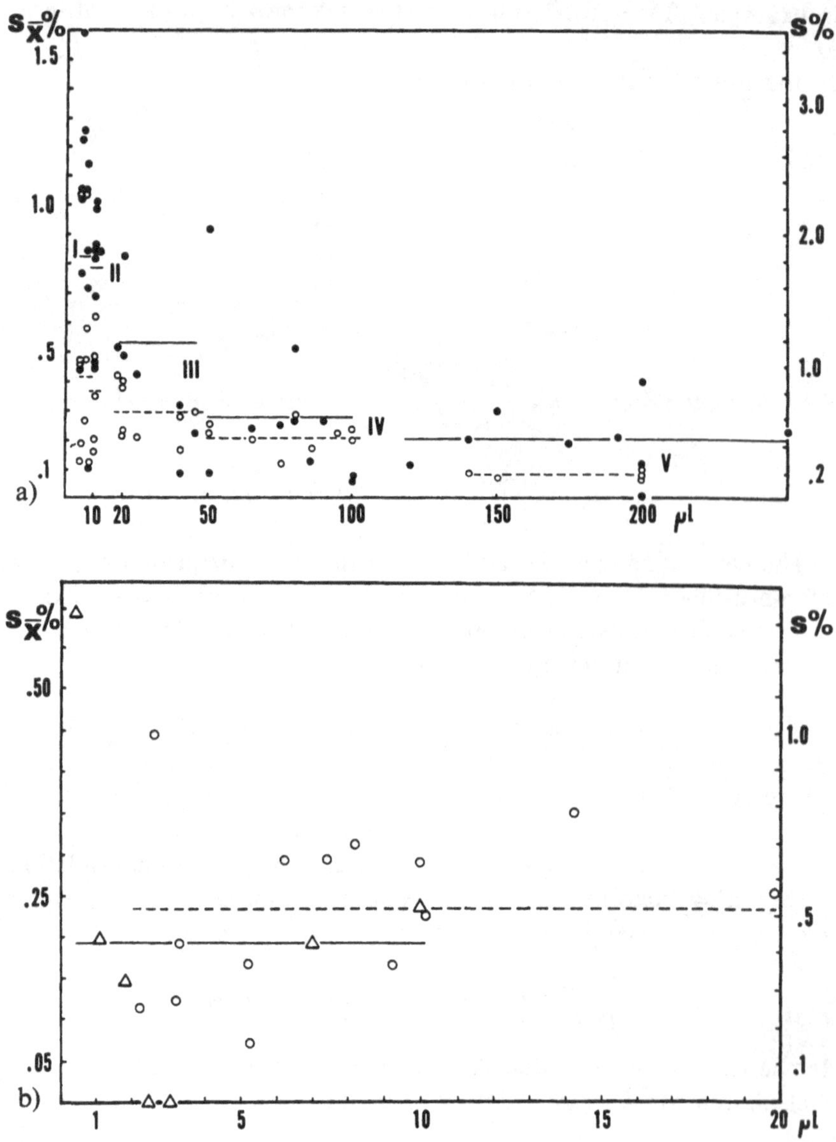

Figure 25. Graphic presentation of calibration results.

Ordinate: s and $s_{\bar{x}}$ in per cent volume. Abscissa: pipet volume in μl; (a) Glass constriction pipets • volumetric calibration; ○ colorimetric calibration. The horizontal lines (solid line gravimetric, dashed line colorimetric) indicate the mean values for the pipets grouped I–V. I. Volumes < 9 μl; II. 9–11 μl; III. 18–45 μl; IV. 50–100 μl; V. 140–200 μl, including the data of a 350-μl pipet not on the graph. (b) (Δ) polyethylene capillary pipets (mean value, solid line); ○ polyethylene constriction pipets (mean value, dashed line). The mean value for polyethylene constriction pipets > 20 μl (not on the graph) is around $s_{\bar{x}}(\%) = \pm 0.1$.

THE "OPTICAL TEST"

The so-called "optical test" was introduced by Otto Warburg in 1936 and is based on the fact that reduced nicotinamide-adenine dinucleotides $NADH_2$ and $NADPH_2$ absorb a maximum of light at 340 nm, while the oxidized forms NAD and NADP show no absorption between 300 and 400 nm. Any dehydrogenase reaction in which either NAD or NADP is reduced or $NADH_2$ or $NADPH_2$ oxidized can be measured by recording the increase or decrease, respectively, of the absorbance at 340 nm or a nearby wavelength. At 366 nm, a frequently used wavelength, *e.g.*, the absorbance of NADH (NADPH) is about one-half of that at 340 nm and is sufficient for most methods described in this book.

The molar extinction coefficients of NADH (NADPH) are $\varepsilon = 6.20 \times \times 10^3$ l/mole × cm at 340 nm and $\varepsilon = 3.30 \times 10^3$ l/mole × cm at 366 nm. This means that 1 mole of NADH (or NADPH) dissolved in 1 liter reduces the transmitted light intensity with 1 cm light path by $\log I_0/I = A = 6.20 \times 10^3$ at 340 nm and by $A = 3.30 \times 10^3$ at 366 nm. The consumption of nicotinamide-adenine dinucleotides can easily be calculated from the changes in absorbance measured in the photometer at 340 or 366 nm.

The measurement of lactate dehydrogenase is an example of the direct or "simple" optical test:

$$\text{pyruvate} + \text{NADH} + \text{H}^+ \rightleftharpoons \text{lactate} + \text{NAD}^+$$

where the rate of oxidation or reduction of the nicotinamide-adenine dinucleotide when measured from left to right, or from right to left, respectively, becomes a measure of the activity of LDH.

The optical test can also be applied to measure an enzyme reaction which is independent of NAD or NADP by "coupling" the reaction with a dehydrogenase system. The determination of the activity of glutamate-pyruvate transaminase (GPT) is an example. GPT catalyzes the reaction

$$\text{alanine} + \text{2-oxoglutarate} \rightleftharpoons \text{pyruvate} + \text{glutamate}$$

In the reaction proceeding from left to right the rate of formation of pyruvate is measured with an "indicator" reaction catalyzed by lactate dehydrogenase (LDH). NADH and an excess of LDH are added to the assay mixture and the reaction will proceed

$$\text{pyruvate} + \text{NADH} + \text{H}^+ \xrightleftharpoons{\text{(LDH)}} \text{lactate} + \text{NAD}^+$$

For each mole of alanine converted into pyruvate by GPT, one mole of NADH is oxidized by LDH, and the rate of decrease in absorbance becomes the parameter for the activity of GPT.

The optical test is not restricted to the coupling of two enzyme reactions, and methods are in use in which the enzyme reaction to be determined and the indicator enzyme reaction are linked by a third or auxiliary enzyme reaction. For an example see creatine phosphokinase (CPK) on page 165. It is logical that the auxiliary enzyme and the indicator enzyme have to be added well in excess to ensure that their activities do not become the limiting factors in the overall reaction.

The optical test can also be applied to determine metabolites, such as pyruvate, lactate and 2-oxoglutarate. While the rate of the substrate turnover is measured in activity determinations, the quantitative consumption is measured in metabolite determinations (example: see Figure 26).

Exact directions for the optical test are given with the description of the various methods. At this point, however, some general remarks will be made.

Unless turbid enzyme solutions, *e.g.*, uncentrifuged homogenates, are used in a test, the reaction can be followed by incubating directly in a cuvette and by continuous recording of the absorbance. Flow-through cuvette holders or thermospacers for the sample compartment, connected

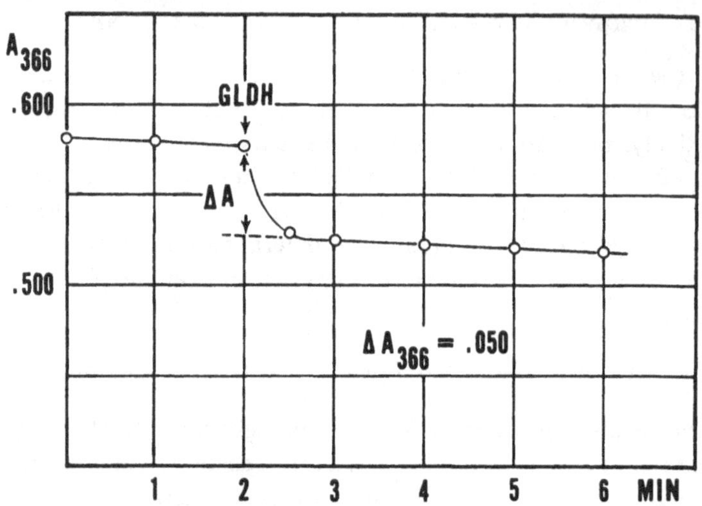

Figure 26. Graphic determination of ΔA in metabolite assays.
Example: 2-oxoglutarate in blood. Experimental conditions: see page 115. The absorbance is plotted over the time in minutes. It is frequently observed that the absorbance decrease does not stop but continues creeping. The exact ΔA is then determined by extrapolation to the start of the reaction (addition of GLDH).

to a cycling thermostat, must be employed in order to achieve rigid temperature control. Enzyme reactions have a temperature coefficient of about 2, which means that an increase in temperature of 10°C doubles the activity, or an increase of 1°C only increases the activity by 10%.

Reagents for an enzyme determination with the optical test are best pipetted directly into the cuvette. All solutions, including serum (or tissue extract), with the exception of the substrate solution, are mixed in the cuvette. Serum and tissue extracts contain small amounts of substrate which react with consumption of NADH (NADPH); when no further change in absorbance is observed (see Figure 27) the enzyme reaction is started by adding the substrate. The absorbance is then read in precisely timed intervals (stop watch), generally 1 minute, and entered into a coordinate system (ordinate: absorbance; abscissa: time in minutes). The use of a recorder simplifies the measurements. The absorbance change per minute (ΔA/min.) should not exceed 0.03–0.04. ΔA/min. is then obtained from the straight part of the curve (Figure 27). As the consumption of NADH (NADPH) continues, the curve tends to flatten.

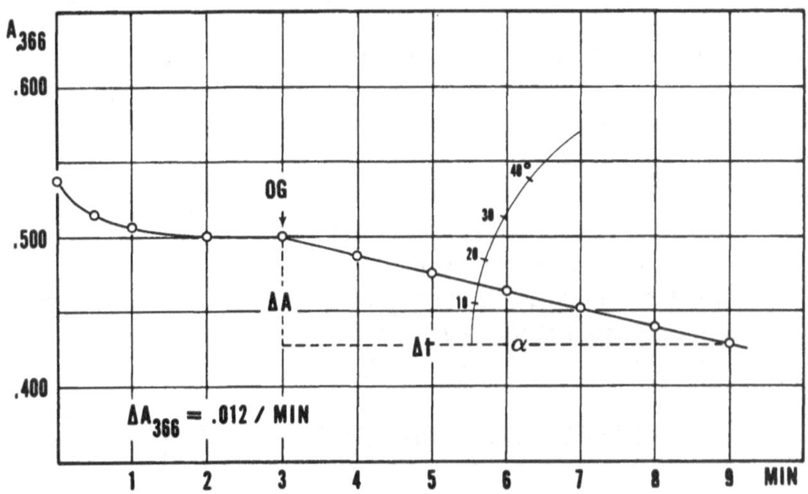

Figure 27. Graphic determination of ΔA/min. in enzyme assays.
Example: glutamate oxaloacetate transaminase (GOT) in serum. Experimental conditions: see page 135. The cuvette is filled with the assay mixture and serum, omitting 2-oxoglutarate (OG). The absorbance decreases because certain serum metabolites react with serum enzymes with NADH consumption. When the absorbance does not decrease further, the reaction is started by adding 2-oxoglutarate. The absorbance is read at one minute intervals for 5–10 minutes and plotted over the time. ΔA/min. is obtained from the straight line drawn through the points. Instead of ΔA/min., tan α × can be used for the calculation (see page 44).

Automatic cuvette changers are available, for example, for the Zeiss spectrophotometer, the Gilford spectrophotometer and the Eppendorf photometer, and these permit simultaneous measurements of four or six samples. To avoid scratching of the glass windows, plastic stirring rods (page 26) are used for mixing in microcuvettes.

Blanks for optical tests

Optical tests generally do not require a reagent blank. The absorbance scale is adjusted to zero either with a water-filled cuvette in the light path, or simply by measuring "against air" (no cuvette in the light path). With the sample cuvette in the light path, the absorbance should read between 0.5 and 0.8. In some instances the enzyme solution itself may have a high self-absorption (*e.g.*, icteric serum, a comparatively large volume of serum in certain tests, a slightly turbid tissue extract) and with the scale adjusted to zero against water or air, absorbances exceeding 0.8 may be encountered with the sample in the light path. One of the following procedures is then recommended:

1. A blank containing buffer is prepared to which the enzyme solution is added in the same proportion as to the reagents in the sample cuvette.
2. If not enough of the enzyme solution is available, NADH-solution is added to water in the blank cuvette in an amount sufficient to bring the difference between blank and sample into the desired absorbance range.
3. Some photometers permit the amplification of the primary photocurrent to be varied within a wide absorbance range. The scale is adjusted to zero against a water blank or against air, and with the sample in the light path the sensitivity is adjusted to bring the absorbance to 0.5–0.8.

CALCULATION OF ENZYME UNITS

In 1961 the Commission on Enzymes of the International Union of Biochemistry recommended a standard unit for all enzymes, which is defined as follows:
"One unit (U) of any enzyme is the amount which will catalyze the transformation of 1 micromole of the substrate per minute under defined conditions."

$$1\ \text{U} = 1\ \mu\text{mole/min.}$$

"With regard to the conditions of measurement, the temperature should be stated and it is suggested that where practicable, it should be 25°C. It will be a great advantage to have a standard temperature which will make it possible to compare the activities of different enzymes. This temperature is high enough to give a reasonable activity, and at the same time low enough to avoid heat denaturation with most enzymes.

"The other conditions should, wherever possible, be optimal, especially with regard to pH and substrate concentration."

In a second revised edition of the report (1964) the temperature suggested was 30°C, a change obviously brought about after it was pointed out that temperature control at 25°C is difficult in hot climates. It is unfortunate that this change was suggested after the standard unit, which included the temperature of 25°C, had been accepted by many investigators and laboratories, and a number of extensive studies had been undertaken to establish "normal values" for enzyme activities in serum. Whatever the outcome of the continuing discussion about the temperature might be, it is now imperative that the temperature at which the enzyme determination was performed be stated.

In my own laboratory, we measure at 25°C, although cooling with tap water is sometimes not sufficient during the hot summer months. But by leading the tap water through a coil immersed in an ice bath before it reaches the thermostat, this difficulty is easily overcome.

In clinical chemistry enzyme activities in body fluids are related to a volume of 1 ml. To avoid inconveniently small numerical values, the results are expressed in milliunits (mU) per ml:

$$\text{mU/ml} = \text{m}\mu\text{moles substrate transformed/min} \times \text{ml}$$

Some clinical chemists prefer one liter as a reference volume and express the activity in U/liter. Numerically "U per liter" and "mU per ml" are identical. The activity of enzymes in tissue is expressed per unit dry weight, fresh weight or protein.

Units of enzyme activity are calculated with reference to a reaction product. The calculation can be based on a "standard" by preparing a solution with an exactly known concentration of the reaction product. An aliquot of the standard solution is treated and measured together with the sample. A standard is not required if the molar extinction coefficient ε of a reaction product is known at a given wavelength as, *e.g.*, for NADH and NADPH.

A. Calculation based on a standard

$$\frac{A_{sample}}{A_{standard}} \times [\text{standard}] \times 10^6 \times \frac{1}{t} = \text{mU/ml}$$

[] = concentration of the standard in moles/1
t = reaction time in minutes.

B. Calculation based on the molar extinction coefficient

a. With the absorbance

$$\frac{A}{\varepsilon \times d} \times 10^6 \times \frac{1}{t} \times \frac{TV}{SV} = \text{mU/ml}$$

ε = molar extinction coefficient
d = diameter of the cuvette (light path) in cm
TV = total assay volume
SV = sample volume
t = reaction time in minutes

The factor 10^6 converts moles/liter or mmoles/ml into mμmoles/ml.

b. With tan α

When time reaction curves are recorded, the angle (α) between the curve and the abscissa can be used for the calculation of enzyme activity (Figure 27).

In the general formula

$$\frac{\Delta A}{\Delta t} \times \frac{10^6}{\varepsilon \times d} \times \frac{TV}{SV} = \text{mU/ml}$$

$\frac{\Delta A}{\Delta t}$ can be substituted:

$$\tan \alpha = \frac{\Delta A}{\Delta t} \times \frac{L_{A=1}}{V_p}; \text{ or } \frac{\Delta A}{\Delta t} = \tan \alpha \times \frac{V_p}{L_{A=1}}$$

V_p = speed of the recording paper in cm/min
$L_{A=1}$ = length in cm to which A = 1.000 is spread;

hence:

$$\tan \alpha \times \frac{V_p}{L_{A=1}} \times \frac{10^6}{\varepsilon \times d} \times \frac{TV}{SV} = \text{mU/ml}$$

Molar extinction coefficient for NADH and NADPH:

3.3×10^3 1/mole $\times$ cm at 366 nm
6.2×10^3 1/mole $\times$ cm at 340 nm
6.0×10^3 1/mole $\times$ cm at 334 nm

Factors to convert other enzyme units into mU/ml are given in Table I:

Table I

Enzyme	Units According to	Factor to Convert into mU/ml
NAD- and NADP-dependent enzyme reactions	Wroblewski	0.48
	Bücher	18.2
	Amelung-Horn	16.7
	Holzer	0.91
	Wolfson-Williams-Ashman	0.0167
phosphohexose isomerase*	Bruns-Hinsberg	0.744
5-phosphoribose isomerase*	Bruns	16.7
acid phosphatase*	King-Armstrong	1.8
	Lowry-Bessey	16.7
alkaline phosphatase*	King-Armstrong	1.8
	Bodansky	5.35
	Lowry-Bessey	16.7

* Measured at 37°C.

CALCULATION OF METABOLITE CONCENTRATIONS IN DETERMINATIONS WITH THE OPTICAL TEST

ε = molar extinction coefficient (page 39)
d = diameter of the cuvette (light path) in cm.

1. $\frac{\Delta A}{\varepsilon \times d} = \text{moles/L} = \text{mmoles/ml} = \mu\text{moles}/\mu\text{l}$

2. $\frac{\Delta A}{\varepsilon \times d} \times \text{assay volume } (\mu\text{l}) = \mu\text{moles/assay volume } (\mu\text{l})$

3. $\frac{\Delta A}{\varepsilon \times d} \times 10^3 \times \frac{\text{assay volume}}{\text{volume of sample}} \times \text{dilution} = \mu\text{moles/ml sample}$

4. $\frac{\mu\text{mole}}{\text{ml}} \times \text{mol. weight} = \mu\text{g/ml}.$

5. $\frac{\mu\text{mole}}{\text{ml}} \times \frac{\text{mol. weight}}{10} = \text{mg/100 ml}$

Chapter 4

Chemical Methods

BILIRUBIN

Literature: Jendrassik, L., and P. Grof, Biochem. Z. **297**, 81 (1938); With, T. K., Z. Physiol. Chem. **278**, 122 (1943) (micromethod); Schellong, G., and U. Wende, Arch. Kinderheilk. **162**, 126 (1960) (semimicromethod).

Principle

Bilirubin is converted to azobilirubin by diazotized sulfanilic acid and is measured colorimetrically. Of the two bilirubin fractions in serum—bilirubin-glucuronide and free bilirubin which is loosely bound to proteins—only the former reacts directly, while free bilirubin reacts after being displaced from protein ("indirect bilirubin"). Displacement in this method is achieved with a caffeine–benzoate–acetate reagent. The difference of two measurements—total bilirubin (with caffeine reagent) and "direct bilirubin" (without caffeine reagent)—enables one to calculate "indirect" bilirubin.

Azobilirubin is red in a neutral solution with an absorption maximum at 530 nm and blue in an alkaline solution with an absorption maximum at 605 nm. The absorbance of the blue dye is considerably higher than that of the red dye. Total bilirubin is therefore preferably measured in alkaline solution. Direct bilirubin must be measured in a neutral solution because at alkaline pH some of the free bilirubin is likely to react.

Reagents

A. *Caffeine reagent:* dissolve 0.5 g caffeine, 0.75 g sodium benzoate and 1.25 g sodium acetate, one after the other, in about 8 ml redistilled water and make up to 10 ml. Filter solution and store in refrigerator.
B. *Diazo I:* dissolve 50 mg sulfanilic acid in 0.15 ml conc. HCl (d = 1.19) and add redistilled water to 10 ml.
C. *Diazo II:* dissolve 25 mg sodium nitrite in 5 ml redistilled water. Store solution B and C in refrigerator.
D. *Diazo reagent:* just before use mix 1 ml (B) with 0.025 ml (C). This reagent is stable for only 30 minutes.
E. *Alkaline tartrate solution:* dissolve 3.5 g K-Na-tartrate and 1 g sodium hydroxide in redistilled water and make up to 10 ml.

Procedure

Total bilirubin

Required amount of serum: 2 × 25 μl
Pipet into a micro test tube

25 μl serum
100 μl caffeine reagent (A)

Mix with vibrator and add

25 μl diazo reagent (D)

Mix and after exactly 10 minutes add

100 μl tartrate solution (E)

Mix and after 5 minutes read absorbance at 605 nm or nearby wavelength (*e.g.*, 578 nm) against a blank which contains 25 μl redistilled water instead of diazo reagent (D).

Direct bilirubin

Required amount of serum: 2 × 25 μl
Pipet into a micro test tube

25 μl serum
200 μl 0.9% saline
25 μl diazo reagent (D)

Mix with vibrator and after exactly 5 minutes read absorbance at

530 nm or nearby wavelength (*e.g.*, 546 nm) against a blank which contains 25 μl redistilled water instead of diazo reagent (D).

Calculation

The calculation factors given are valid only for measurement of total bilirubin at 578 nm and direct bilirubin at 546 nm and for the recommended volumes. For measurements at different wavelengths and/or with deviating volumes, recalculation of the factors is essential (see page 114).

Total bilirubin:

$$A_{578} \times 9 = \text{mg total bilirubin/100 ml serum}$$

Direct bilirubin:

$$A_{546} \times 12 = \text{mg direct bilirubin/100 ml serum}$$

Indirect bilirubin:

total bilirubin–direct bilirubin.

The factors are based on the molar extinction coefficient of pure bilirubin in chloroform at 453 nm, $\varepsilon = 60100$. Bilirubin standard solutions are very unstable and are therefore unsuitable for routine controls. It is recommended, however, that the calculation factors be determined according to the procedure described below and that the standardization be repeated once every month or so.

Preparation of bilirubin standards:

1. Determination of the purity of bilirubin preparations [Richterich, R., Klin. Wochschr. **41**, 778 (1963)]:
   Dry bilirubin in a desiccator in the dark. Weigh out exactly 10 mg and dissolve with chloroform to 100 ml. For the determination dilute 1:10 with chloroform, concentration = 1 mg bilirubin/100 ml. This solution is stable for 30 minutes only. Avoid exposure to light. Measure absorbance in a 10-mm cuvette at 453 nm (maximum of absorbance) against chloroform as blank (= $A_{453}^{prep.}$). The molar extinction coefficient of pure bilirubin in chloroform at 453 nm equals $\varepsilon = 60100$ (recommendation on uniform bilirubin standard: Clin. Chem. **8**, 405, 1962). Molecular weight of bilirubin = 584.7.
   First calculate the theoretical absorbance of pure bilirubin (= $A_{453}^{theor.}$).

$$A_{453}^{theor.} = \frac{\varepsilon \times C\,(g\%) \times 1 \times 10}{\text{mol. wt.}} = \frac{60100 \times 0.001 \times 10}{584.7} = 1.03$$

and then the purity of the preparation in per cent

$$\% \text{ purity} = \frac{A_{453}^{\text{prep.}} \times 100}{A_{453}^{\text{theor.}}} = \frac{A_{453}^{\text{prep.}} \times 100}{1.03} = A_{453}^{\text{prep.}} \times 97$$

If measurements are made with the Eppendorf photometer, a 436 nm filter is to be used: $\varepsilon = 56\,800$

$$\% \text{ purity} = \frac{A_{436}^{\text{prep.}} \times 100}{0.973} = A_{436}^{\text{prep.}} \times 103$$

2. Bilirubin standard solution: 10 mg/100 ml (Schellong, G., and U. Wende: Klin. Wochschr. **38**, 703, 1960): dissolve exactly 40 mg pure bilirubin (or more according to purity) with 1% sodium carbonate to exactly 50 ml. To 13.9 ml of a commercial standard serum *free of bilirubin,* add 2.0 ml bilirubin solution and 0.1 ml 25% acetic acid.

   Bilirubin concentration = 10 mg/100 ml. (If a bilirubin-free serum is not available, use a normal, nonicteric serum. Determine the bilirubin content in a mixture of 13.9 ml serum, 2.0 ml 1% sodium carbonate and 0.1 ml acetic acid and subtract from serum with bilirubin standard added.)

   The bilirubin standard serum is used to determine the molar extinction coefficients of azobilirubin at the selected wavelength between 560 and 605 nm for the determination of total bilirubin and at the selected wavelength between 530 and 555 nm for the determination of direct bilirubin.

$$\varepsilon = A \times \frac{\text{mol. wt.}}{C\,(g\%) \times 1 \times 10} \times \frac{\text{total volume}}{\text{vol. of stand sol.}}$$

$$\varepsilon = A \times \frac{584.7}{0.01 \times 1 \times 10} \times \frac{250}{25} = A \times 58470.$$

Example

Method for total bilirubin: measurements at 578 nm
Found: $A_{578} = 1.111$
$\varepsilon = 1.111 \times 58470 = 64960$

Calculation

mg bilirubin (total)/100 ml serum =

$$A_{578} \times \frac{\text{mol. wt.}}{\varepsilon \times 1 \times 10} \times 1000 \times \frac{\text{total volume}}{\text{volume of serum sample}} =$$

$$A_{578} \times \frac{584.7}{64960 \times 10} \times 1000 \times \frac{250}{25} = A \times 9.$$

Method for direct bilirubin; measurement at 546 nm
Found: $A_{546} = 0.833$
$\varepsilon = 0.833 \times 58470 = 48705$

Calculation

mg bilirubin (direct)/100 ml serum =

$$A_{546} \times \frac{584.7}{48705 \times 1 \times 10} \times 1000 \times \frac{250}{25} = A_{546} \times 12.$$

Normal values in serum:

total bilirubin up to 1 mg/100 ml
direct bilirubin up to 0.25 mg/100 ml.

CALCIUM

Method 1: with murexide as indicator

Literature: Elliott, W. E., J. Biol. Chem. **197**, 641 (1952); Siegmund, P., and H. J. Dulce, Z. Physiol. Chem. **320**, 149 (1960) (micromethod).

Principle

Calcium can be titrated directly in serum with ethylenediaminotetraacetate (EDTA). In strongly alkaline solution and with murexide as indicator, magnesium does not interfere. The end point of the titration (color change from red to violet) can be determined photometrically.

Reagents

Glassware and reagents must be free of calcium. Use water redistilled from a quartz apparatus or deionized water. Store solutions in polyethylene bottles.

A. *NaOH* 0.1N
B. *Murexide solution:* 30 mg% in redistilled water
C. *Ethylenediaminotetraacetate* 2.5×10^{-3}M: dissolve in redistilled water 0.73 g of the free acid or 0.93 g of the disodium salt × H_2O or 0.95 g of the tetrasodium salt and make up to 1000 ml.

Procedure

Required amount of serum or plasma: 100 µl
Pipet into a 40-mm *macro*cuvette

9 ml redistilled water
2 ml NaOH (A)
0.3 ml murexide (B)
0.1 ml serum

Mix well with plastic spatula and adjust absorbance (at 480 or 590 nm) to 0.3–0.5 either by reading against an appropriate neutral filter or by partial compensation of the photoelectric current (if the instrument is so equipped). Any microburet with 1 µl or 2 µl divisions is suitable for the titration. Connect a narrow polyethylene tube to the tip of the buret and fill bubble-free with EDTA solution. Dip the free end of tubing into the solution to be titrated; make sure that the tubing does not reach into the light path (!). Deliver EDTA solution slowly in approximately 10-µl portions. After adding each portion, mix well and read absorbance and μl EDTA delivered. The absorbance decreases linearly until the end point is reached. Deliver an excess three 10–μl portions.

On graph paper plot absorbance over μl EDTA consumed. At the end point, the curve has a break. Draw a straight line through the points of each segment of the curve. The intersection indicates the exact end point of the titration. Read μl EDTA consumed from the abscissa. For each series of measurements prepare and process a blank containing redistilled water, NaOH and murexide.

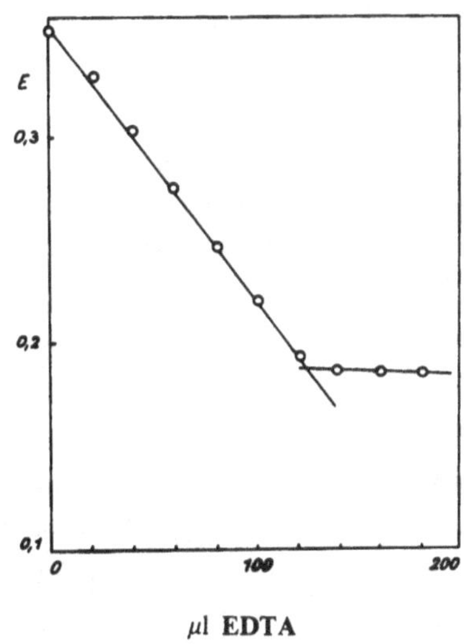

Figure 28. Graphic determination of the exact end point of the Ca-titration with EDTA; see text.

Calculation

$$(\mu l\ EDTA_{sample} - \mu l\ EDTA_{blank}) \times 0.1 = mg\ calcium/100\ ml\ serum$$

Method 2: with calcein as indicator

Literature: Dichl, H., and J. L. Ellingboe, Anal. Chem. **28**, 822 (1956); Beckman Technical Bulletin # 6071 C (micromethod).

Principle

The principle is the same as described above (Method 1) but calcein (condensation product of iminoacetic acid and fluorescin) serves as the indicator. Calcein forms a fluorescent yellowish-green color complex with Ca-ions. The color changes to a nonfluorescent orange-red when the total calcium is bound by EDTA.

Reagents

Store all reagents in polyethylene bottles.

A. *KOH* 1.25N: dissolve 7.0 g KOH and 50 mg KCN in redistilled water and dilute to 100 ml.

B. *Indicator solution:* dissolve 25 mg calcein in 100 ml 0.25N NaOH.

C. *Ethylenediaminotetraacetate* 0.02N: in a 100-ml volumetric flask dissolve 372 mg of the disodium salt × H_2O in redistilled water and fill to the mark.

D. *Calcium standard* 5 meq/liter: dissolve 25.0 mg dry $CaCO_3$ in 0.6 ml 0.1N HCl in a small glass beaker. Boil off excess HCl. Allow to cool, transfer into a 100 ml volumetric flask, and fill to the mark with redistilled water.

Procedure

Required amount of serum: 20 μl
Pipet into a microtitrator

20 μl serum
100 μl KOH (A)
10 μl indicator (B)

Mix and titrate with EDTA. In addition prepare and titrate a standard with 20 μl Ca standard (D) instead of serum and a blank with 20 μl redistilled water instead of serum. Use the same pipet for serum, standard and water.

The end point of the titration can be recognized either by the appearance of the orange-red color or by the disappearance of the yellowish-green fluorescence. The fluorescence can best be seen in ultraviolet light (emission maximum 3600 Å). The Beckman Spinco microtitrator 153 is highly recommended for the titration (see page 27).

Calculation

$$\frac{\mu l\ EDTA_{sample} - \mu l\ EDTA_{blank}}{\mu l\ EDTA_{stand.} - \mu l\ EDTA_{blank}} \times 5 = \text{meq calcium/liter serum}$$

$$\text{meq calcium/liter} \times 2 = \text{mg calcium/100 ml}$$

Normal values in serum:

8.5–10.5 mg calcium/100 ml = 4.25–5.25 meq/liter.

IRON

All glassware, polyethylene vessels, bottles and pipets must be carefully washed with HCl diluted 1:2 and rinsed with redistilled water.

Method 1: without deproteinization

Literature: Lauber, K., Z. Klin. Chem. **3**, 96 (1965).

Principle

Serum-iron is separated from transferrin by the anionic wetting agent Teepol, reduced with dithionite, and determined photometrically as a red color complex of bathophenanthroline disulfonate; deproteinization is not necessary.

Reagents

A. *Teepol 710* (Shell Chemical Company)

B. *Sodium dithionite* ($Na_2S_2O_4$)

C. *$MgSO_4$ solution* 1%: dissolve 1 g $MgSO_4 \times 7\ H_2O$ in 100 ml redistilled water.

D. *NaOH* 3%: dissolve 3 g NaOH in 100 ml redistilled water.

E. *Teepol reagent*, iron-free: dissolve 0.5 g dithionite (B) in 10 ml $MgSO_4$ solution (C) and immediately add 10 ml Teepol (A), followed by 5 ml NaOH (D). Allow the cloudy mixture to stand for 10–15 minutes, then centrifuge. Iron contained in Teepol is precipitated as $Fe(OH)_2$ together with $Mg(OH)_2$. Transfer supernatant into a glass beaker and adjust pH with glacial acetic acid to 5.4–6.2. Store reagent in several small polyethylene bottles, each containing the amount for one day's work. Fill bottles to the rim, close tightly and store at 4°C. The reagent is stable for about seven weeks. Air gradually diminishes the reducing efficiency.

F. *Bathophenanthroline solution:* dissolve 100 mg disodium bathophenantroline-disulfonate in 10 ml redistilled water. The solution is stable indefinitely.

G. *Iron standard:* dilute a commercial iron standard with redistilled water to 100 μg Fe/100 ml.

Procedure

Required amount of serum: 50 μl (clear serum)
Pipet into a 10-mm microcuvette

50 μl serum
140 μl Teepol reagent (E)
1 μl color reagent (F)

Mix thoroughly with polyethylene stirrer. The color is fully developed after 10 seconds. Read absorbance at wavelength between 500 and 550 nm against water. Together with the serum prepare a blank with 50 μl redistilled water and a standard with 50 μl iron standard (G) instead of serum.

Lipemic serum is allowed to stand at room temperature for 15 minutes after Teepol reagent (E) has been added. The chylomicrons dissolve in the presence of the wetting agent and the mixture becomes clear. Then color reagent (F) is added. Use the same pipet for serum sample, standard and water. Beer's law is valid up to 1000 μg Fe/100 ml. With an absorbance > 0.4 add 2 μl of the color reagent (F).

Calculation

$$\frac{A_{\text{sample}} - A_{\text{blank}}}{A_{\text{standard}} - A_{\text{blank}}} \times 100 = \mu\text{g Fe/100 ml serum}$$

Normal values: 50–180 μg Fe/100 ml serum.

The macromethod (Lauber) was adapted for microliter analysis in the author's laboratory in Chicago. At that time Teepol 710 was not available in the United States. Shell Chemical Company suggested the use of Teepol 610, which is less concentrated. It was observed that with Teepol 610 the time for full color development was prolonged to 5 minutes. If Teepol 610 is used, the test mixtures are prepared in polyethylene micro test tubes and transferred into microcuvettes after 15 minutes or more (the color is stable).

Iron-binding capacity

Reagents

A. *Ferric chloride solution:* 2.5 mg/100 ml redistilled water.

B. *Basic magnesium carbonate*

Procedure

Required amount of serum: 50 μl
Pipet into polyethylene micro test tube

50 μl serum

100 μl $FeCl_3$ (A)

Mix with vibrator and after 5 minutes add

appr. 5 mg $MgCO_3$ **(B)**

Mix and allow to stand for 30 minutes. During this time resuspend precipitate (vibrator) about every 5 minutes. Centrifuge to remove $MgCO_3$ and excess iron absorbed as hydroxide. Determine iron in 50 μl of the clear supernatant with Method 1.

Calculation of iron-binding capacity

$$\frac{A_{sample} - A_{blank}}{A_{standard} - A_{blank}} \times 300 = \mu g\ Fe/100\ ml\ serum$$

Normal values in serum: 280–400 μg Fe/100 ml

Method 2: with deproteinization

Literature: Zak, B., and J. W. Landers, Am. J. Clin. Pathol. **29**, 590 (1958); Neth, R., H. Schäfer, D. Goschenhofer, and E. Laak, Klin. Wochschr. **41**, 1089 (1963) (micromethod).

Principle

Serum iron is separated from transferrin by acid hydrolysis, reduced with ascorbic acid after deproteinization, and determined photometrically as red color complex of bathophenanthroline disulfonate.

Reagents

A. *HCl* 1.0N

B. *Trichloroacetic acid* 3M: dissolve 49 g trichloroacetic acid in redistilled water and make up to 100 ml.

C. *Ascorbic acid solution* 10%

D. *Color reagent:* dissolve 30.0 mg disodium bathophenanthroline disulfonate in 100 ml 4.0M acetate buffer, pH 4.6.

E. *Iron standard:* dilute a commercial iron standard with redistilled water to 250 μg Fe/100 ml.

Procedure

Required amount of serum: 200 μl
Pipet into a micro test tube

200 μl serum
100 μl HCl (A)

Mix with vibrator and allow to stand at room temperature for 30 minutes. Then add

50 μl TCA (B)

Mix; allow to stand for a few minutes and centrifuge. Pipet into a micro test tube

200 μl supernatant
10 μl ascorbic acid (C)

Mix and allow to stand at room temperature for 5 minutes, then add

100 μl color reagent (D)

Mix and read absorbance after 5 minutes or more at 500–550 nm in a 10-mm microcuvette against water. Prepare and process a blank with 200 μl redistilled water and a standard with 200 μl iron standard (E) instead of serum.
Use the same pipet for serum, water and standard.

Calculation

$$\frac{A_{\text{sample}} - A_{\text{blank}}}{A_{\text{standard}} - A_{\text{blank}}} \times 250 = \mu g \text{ Fe/100 ml serum}$$

Normal values:

men	90–140 μg/100 ml serum
women	80–120 μg/100 ml serum

Calculations can also be made with a factor obtained from a calibration curve. If not enough serum is available, reduce all volumes to $\frac{1}{2}$; careful vertical adjustment of the cuvettes in the light beam becomes essential (see page 9). If a serum copper analysis is to be made at the same time, double the amount of serum, HCl and TCA and use 200 μl of the supernatant after deproteinization (see below).

COPPER

Literature: Zack, B., and J. W. Landers, Am. J. Clin. Pathol. **29**, 590 (1958); Neth, R., K. H. Schäfer, D. Goschenhofer, and E. Laak, Klin. Wochschr. **41**, 1089 (1963) (micromethod).

Principle

Copper in serum is separated from ceruloplasmin and other proteins by acid hydrolysis, deproteinized, reduced with ascorbic acid, and determined photometrically as brownish-yellow color complex of bathocuproine-disulfonate.

Reagents

A. *HCl* 1.0N
B. *Trichloroacetic acid* 3M: dissolve 49 g trichloroacetic acid in redistilled water to form 100 ml.
C. *Ascorbic acid solution* 10%
D. *Color reagent:* dissolve 30 mg disodium bathocuproine disulfonate in 100 ml 3.3M sodium acetate solution.
E. *Copper standard:* dilute a commercial copper standard with redistilled water to 250 μg Cu/100 ml.

Procedure

Required amount of serum: 200 μl
Pipet into micro test tube

	200 μl serum
	100 μl HCl (A)
Mix with vibrator and allow to stand at room temperature for 30 minutes. Then add	
	50 μl TCA (B)
Mix, allow to stand for a few minutes and centrifuge. Pipet into a micro test tube	
	200 μl supernatant
	10 μl ascorbic acid (C)
Mix and allow to stand at room temperature for 5 minutes. Then add	
	100 μl color reagent (D)

Mix and read absorbance after 5 minutes or more at 420–440 nm in a 10-mm cuvette against water. Prepare and process a blank with 200 μl redistilled water and a standard with 200 μl copper standard (E) instead of serum.
Use the same pipet for serum, water and standard.

Calculation

$$\frac{A_{\text{sample}} - A_{\text{blank}}}{A_{\text{standard}} - A_{\text{blank}}} \times 250 = \mu\text{g Cu/100 ml serum}$$

Normal values: 90–130 μg/100 ml serum

Calculations can also be made with a factor obtained from a standard curve. If not enough serum is available, reduce all volumes to $\frac{1}{2}$; careful vertical adjustment of the cuvettes in the light beam then becomes essential (see page 9). If serum iron is to be determined at the same time, double the amount of serum, HCl and TCA and use 200 μl of deproteinized supernatant for iron analysis (see above).

KETONE BODIES

Literature: Hansen, O., Scand. J. Clin. Lab. Invest. **11**, 259 (1959) (micromethod).

Principle

The blood analysis for ketone bodies, *i.e.*, acetoacetic acid, β-hydroxybutyric acid and acetone, involves the following steps: (1) conversion of acetoacetic acid and β-hydroxybutyric acid into acetone with chromosulfuric acid; (2) distillation of acetone; (3) formation of acetonehydrazone with 2,4-dinitrophenylhydrazine, and decomposition of other hydrazones formed and of excess 2,4-dinitrophenylhydrazine with NaOH; (4) extraction of acetonehydrazone with carbon tetrachloride and colorimetric determination at 349 nm.

Reagents

A. *Sodium tungstate solution,* 10%: dissolve 25 g $Na_2WO_4 \times 2\ H_2O$ in 250 ml redistilled water.
B. *H_2SO_4* 0.66N: into a 1500 ml round-bottomed flask, pipet 250 ml 0.66N H_2SO_4 (prepared from conc. H_2SO_4) and 75 ml redistilled water. Heat over a flame and concentrate the solution to approximately 250 ml, boiling not less than 30 minutes. After cooling, the acid is adjusted to exactly 0.66N, with a factor not exceeding $\pm$ 0.01.
C. *Chromosulfuric acid:* into a 1500-ml round-bottomed flask, pipet 152 ml redistilled water and carefully add 80.0 ml conc. H_2SO_4 (spec. gravity 1.84) and 80.0 ml of an exactly 5% (w/v) $K_2Cr_2O_7$-solution in redistilled water. Proceed as directed in B and concentrate the solution to 240 ml. The $H_2SO_4/K_2Cr_2O_7$ ratio has to be exact. According to Hansen sulfuric acid and chromate, even of highest purity, contain substances which increase the blank value significantly but which are eliminated by boiling. It is therefore essential to follow precisely the directions for preparing (B) and (C).
D. *Carbon tetrachloride*
E. *2,4-dinitrophenylhydrazine solution* 0.1% (w/v) in 2N HCl
F. *NaOH* 0.5N

Procedure

Required amount of blood: 25–200 μl, heparinized. Results are understated when the blood is even partially clotted. Blood may be drawn directly from the vein into micro test tubes covered with a layer of heparin. (Rinse test tubes with heparin solution and allow to dry inverted on filter paper.)

Pipet into a 2-ml centrifuge tube

Pipet into a 2-ml centrifuge tube	0.025–0.200 ml blood 1.575–1.400 ml H_2O 1.600 ml total volume
Mix with vibrator and add	0.200 ml tungstate (A)
Mix and add	0.200 ml H_2SO_4 (B)
Mix well and allow the covered tube to stand for 10 minutes. Centrifuge for 15 minutes at 3000 rpm. Pipet into distilling apparatus (Figure 29)	1.0 ml clear supernatant 14.0 ml H_2O 1.5 ml chromosulfuric acid (C)
Start distillation and continue until the mixture is condensed to approximately 2 ml. Dilute distillate with redistilled water to exactly 15.0 ml. Pipet into a glass-stoppered 25-ml cylinder	3.0 ml diluted distillate 2.0 ml dinitrophenylhydrazine (E) 10.0 ml CCl_4 (D)

Shake intensively for 5 minutes. Transfer mixture into a separatory funnel. After separation return CCl_4-phase to the cylinder. Rinse separatory funnel with water. Return CCl_4-phase to the separatory funnel, add 10 ml redistilled water and shake. Return CCl_4-phase to the cylinder, add 3 ml NaOH (F) and shake for 3 minutes. Transfer solution into a clean, dry separatory funnel. After separation read absorbance of the CCl_4-phase in 10-mm cuvettes against CCl_4 (D) at 349 nm. Reagent blank: use 3 ml redistilled water instead of diluted distillate, add dinitrophenylhydrazine (E) and CCl_4 (B) and proceed as directed.

Acetone standard: acetone solution with 4.0 mg acetone/100 ml redistilled water. Use 0.200 ml of this instead of blood, add tungstate (A) and H_2SO_4 (B) and proceed as directed.

Calculation

$$\frac{(A_{sample} - A_{blank}) \times 0.008 \times 100}{(A_{standard} - A_{blank}) \times B} = \text{mg ketone bodies, expressed as acetone per 100 ml blood}$$

A_{sample} = absorption of blood sample
A_{blank} = absorption of reagent blank
$A_{standard}$ = absorption of acetone standard
B = blood volume in ml.

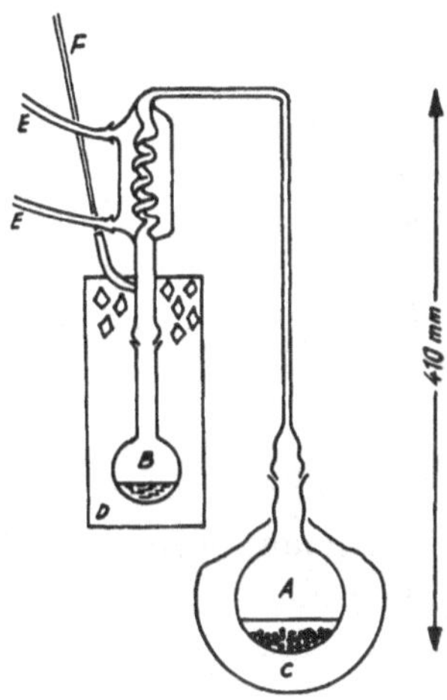

Figure 29. Microdistillation apparatus according to O. Hansen.

A. distillation flask,
B. receiving flask,
C. electric heating jacket,
D. ice bath,
E. tubes for water cooling,
F. reflux tube.

Available from Struers, Copenhagen, Denmark.

CREATINE

Literature: Abelin, J., and J. Raaflaub, Biochem. Z. **323**, 382 (1952–53).

Principle

Creatine reacts with diacetyl and α-naphthol in alkaline solution to form a red dye which is determined photometrically.

Reagents

A. *NaOH* 1.5N
B. *Diacetyl stock solution* 1% in redistilled water
C. *Diacetyl working solution* 0.05%: shortly before use dilute 1 ml stock solution with 19 ml redistilled water.
D. *Alkaline α-naphthol solution* 1%: dissolve 10 mg α-naphthol in 1 ml 1.5N NaOH (A). Prepare shortly before use.
E. *Metaphosphoric acid* 5%: prepare shortly before use.

Procedure

Required amount of serum: 100 μl
Pipet into a micro test tube (1)

	100 μl serum 100 μl metaphosphoric acid (E)
Mix with vibrator and centrifuge at high speed. Transfer supernatant with a polyethylene pipet having a long thin tip into a micro test tube with a mark at 400 μl (2). Add to the precipitate in (1)	
	100 μl metaphosphoric acid
Suspend precipitate by vigorous vibration. Centrifuge at high speed and add supernatant to (2). Repeat extraction once and add supernatant to (2). Fill with metaphosphoric acid to the 400 μl mark. Mix with vibrator. Pipet into a micro test tube	
	50 μl α-naphthol (D) 50 μl combined supernatants 25 μl diacetyl (C) 125 μl redistilled water

Mix vigorously with vibrator (access of air is essential) and allow to stand in an open tube for 30 minutes. Read absorbance in a 10-mm microcuvette at 530 nm or nearby wavelength against a reagent blank. Reagent blank: 100 μl redistilled water + 300 μl metaphosphoric acid. Use 50 μl instead of the combined supernatants in the final assay mixture. The color is stable for about 40 minutes.

With low serum concentrations increase the amount of combined supernatants in the final assay mixture and reduce the amount of water accordingly.

Calculation

Construct a calibration curve with pure creatine. From a standard solution of 2.0 mg creatine/100 ml, prepare a dilution series. To 100 μl of each dilution add 300 μl metaphosphoric acid and use 50 μl in the final assay mixture.

Normal values in serum: 0.8–1.2 mg/100 ml.

CREATININE

Several colorimetric methods to determine serum creatinine have been suggested, none of which is absolutely specific for creatinine. It is left to the investigator to make his choice.

Values obtained with dinitrobenzoic acid (Method 1) are said to be closest to the actual creatinine concentration, but the color is unstable and the reproducibility therefore not very satisfactory.

In Jaffe's technique (Method 2) other reducing substances—ascorbic acid, pyruvate, glucose—react with picric acid but the rate of color development is considerably slower with these unspecific chromogens than with creatinine.

Creatinine can be separated from the unspecific chromogens (Method 3) by adsorption on Lloyd's reagent (purified Fuller's earth); in my experience, however, the elution is not always complete and may vary with the preparation of Lloyd's reagent. A creatinine standard must therefore be treated simultaneously with the serum sample. The method with Lloyd's reagent is time-consuming and therefore disliked in the routine laboratory. Direct serum deproteinization with picric acid (Method 4) seems to eliminate at least some of the interference of the unspecific chromogens. The determination is fast and simple, and the results are comparable to those obtained with Lloyd's reagent. Since erythrocytes contain unspecific chromogens, serum should be free of visible hemolysis.

Method 1: with dinitrobenzoic acid

Literature: Standard Methods of Clinical Chemistry **1**, 55 (1953).

Principle

Creatinine reacts with dinitrobenzoic acid in alkaline solution to form a red color complex which is determined photometrically.

Reagents

A. *Dinitrobenzoic acid solution* 10%: dissolve with heating 1 g 3,5-dinitrobenzoic acid in 2.5 ml 10% sodium carbonate; add 7.5 ml redistilled water and filter.

B. H_2SO_4 1.333N: add 4 ml conc. H_2SO_4 slowly to 100 ml redistilled water. Adjust strength by titration with standardized 1.0N NaOH against phenolphthalein.

C. *Sodium tungstate solution* 20%: store in polyethylene bottle.

D. *NaOH* 2.5N

E. *Creatinine stock solution:* dissolve 10.0 mg anhydrous creatinine in 10 ml 0.1N HCl.

F. *Creatinine working standard:* dilute 200 μl (E) with redistilled water to 10.0 ml (50 μl = 1 μg creatinine).

Procedure

Required amount of serum: 50 μl

Pipet into a micro test tube	50 μl serum 150 μl redistilled water
Add slowly with frequent mixing (vibrator)	25 μl H_2SO_4 (B) 25 μl tungstate (C)
Centrifuge. Transfer into a micro test tube	150 μl clear supernatant 45 μl dinitrobenzoic acid (A) 7.5 μl NaOH (D)

Mix with vibrator and allow to stand *in the dark* at room temperature for 10 minutes. Read absorbance at 500 nm (or nearby wavelength) in 10-mm microcuvette against a blank containing 150 μl redistilled water instead of supernatant in the final assay mixture.

For each series include a standard with 150 μl working standard (F) instead of supernatant in the final assay mixture. Transfer of the solution into a cuvette and reading the absorbance should not take longer than 1 minute because the color begins to fade when exposed to light.

Calculation

The assay mixture contains $\frac{3}{5}$ = 30 μl of 50 μl serum. Amount of creatinine in standard assay mixture = 3 μg.

$$\frac{A_{sample}}{A_{standard}} \times 10.0 = \text{mg creatinine/100 ml serum}$$

If normal or slightly elevated creatinine concentrations are expected dilute working standard further to 1:5 or 1:10; the calculation factor then becomes 2.0 or 1.0 respectively (amount of creatinine in standard assay mixture × 3.333).
Normal values in serum: 0.6–1.05 mg creatinine/100 ml.

Method 2: with picric acid

Literature: Owen, J. A., B. Iggo, F. J. Scandrett, and C. P. Stewart, Biochem. J. **58**, 426 (1954).

Principle

Creatinine is determined in deproteinized serum with Jaffe's reaction, and the red color complex is determined photometrically.

Reagents

A. *Sodium tungstate* 10%

B. H_2SO_4 0.66N

C. *Picric acid* 0.04N: dissolve 916 mg anhydrous picric acid in redistilled water (may be heated) to form 100 ml. Store in the dark.

D. *NaOH* 0.75N

E. *Creatinine stock solution:* dissolve 15.0 mg anhydrous creatinine in 10 ml 0.1N HCl. The solution is stable indefinitely when stored in the refrigerator.

F. *Creatinine working standard:* dilute stock solution 1:100 with redistilled water. Concentration: 1.5 mg/100 ml. A standard control serum may be used instead of the creatinine standard.

Procedure

Required amount of serum: 100 μl
Pipet into a micro test tube

	100 μl serum
	150 μl H_2O
Mix with a vibrator and add	
	50 μl tungstate (A)
Mix and add	
	100 μl H_2SO_4 (B)

Mix and allow to stand for a few minutes. Centrifuge at high speed.
Pipet into a micro test tube

150 μl clear supernatant
50 μl picric acid (C)
50 μl NaOH (D)

Mix with vibrator. After exactly 20 minutes read absorbance in a 10-mm microcuvette at 520–555 nm against a blank with 150 μl water instead of supernatant. Treat standard (F) like the serum sample.

Calculation

$$\frac{A_{\text{sample}}}{A_{\text{standard}}} \times \text{standard (mg/100 ml)} = \text{mg creatinine/100 ml serum}$$

Method 3: with Lloyd's reagent

Literature: see Method 2.

Principle

Creatinine is adsorbed on Fuller's earth (Lloyd's reagent), while other chromogens remain in solution. After centrifuging creatinine is eluted and determined with picric acid.

Reagents

A–F: see Method 2
G. *Oxalic acid:* saturated solution
H. *Lloyd's reagent:* suspend 10 g purified Fuller's earth in 100 ml redistilled water. Test each preparation for its capacity to adsorb creatinine.

Procedure

Deproteinize serum as described in Method 2.

Pipet into a micro test tube

150 μl clear supernatant
100 μl H_2O
25 μl oxalic acid (G)
50 μl Lloyd's reagent (H)

Allow to stand for 10 minutes and mix repeatedly with vibrator. Centrifuge at high speed. Remove supernatant as completely as possible with a polyethylene capillary pipet. Add to precipitate

150 μl H_2O
50 μl picric acid (C)
50 μl NaOH (D)

Allow to stand for 10 minutes and mix repeatedly with vibrator. Make sure that the precipitate is completely suspended by vibration. Centrifuge and after an additional 10 minutes read absorbance as described in Method 2.

Treat a blank (H_2O) and a standard (solution F) together with serum. Normal values in mg/100 ml serum:

without Lloyd's reagent:	men	0.9–1.4
	women	0.8–1.2
with Lloyd's reagent:	men	0.7–1.2
	women	0.5–1.0

Method 4: Direct deproteinization with picric acid

Literature: Popper, H., E. Mandel, and H. Manger, Biochem. Z. **291**, 354 (1937); Schirrmeister, J., H. Willmann, and H. Kiefer, Klin. Wochschr. **41,** 878 (1963).

Principle

Similar to Method 2, but serum is deproteinized with picric acid.

Reagents

A. *Picric acid,* saturated solution: dissolve 1.4 g picric acid in 100 ml hot redistilled water. Cool to room temperature and filter. Store solution in the dark.
B. *NaOH* 10%
C. *Creatinine standard:* see Method 2, E and F.

Procedure

Required amount of serum: 100 μl

Pipet into a micro test tube

300 μl picric acid (A)
100 μl serum

Mix with vibrator. Allow to stand for a few minutes, then centrifuge.
Pipet into a micro test tube

250 μl supernatant
25 μl NaOH (B)

Mix with vibrator. After exactly 20 minutes read absorbance as described in Method 2. Treat a blank (H_2O) and a standard together with serum.

Calculation

See Method 2.
Normal values in mg/100 ml serum:

men 0.6–1.2; mean 0.92
women 0.6–1.1; mean 0.76.

INORGANIC PHOSPHATE

Literature: Lowry, O. H., and J. A. Lopez, J. Biol. Chem. **162**, 421 (1945). For the micromodification see H. Mattenheimer, Acta Biol. Med. Ger. **1**, 405 (1958).

Principle

Phosphate reacts with ammonium molybdate to form ammonium phosphomolybdate, which is reduced to molybdenium blue with ascorbic acid. The determination is made at pH 4. No measurable hydrolysis of acid-labile organic phosphates occurs during the time necessary for analysis.

Reagents

A. *Trichloroacetic acid* (TCA) 8%
B. *Ammonium molybdate:* 1% in redistilled water
C. *Ascorbic acid:* 1% in redistilled water
D. *Acetate buffer* 0.1M, pH 4.0
E. *Sodium acetate* 0.2M
F. *Buffer mixture:* mix 11 parts D with 3 parts E
G. *Phosphate stock solution:* in a 100-ml volumetric flask dissolve 0.4387 g KH_2PO_4 (anhydrous, Sørensen) in redistilled water and fill to the mark; 1ml = 1 mg P.
H. *Phosphate working standard:* dilute stock solution 1:20 with redistilled water; concentration: 5 mg P/100 ml.

Procedure

Required amount of serum: 10 μl
Place micro test tubes in an ice bath.
Pipet into a micro test tube

10 μl serum
20 μl TCA (ice cold)

Mix with vibrator and allow to stand in ice bath for 5 minutes. Centrifuge, pipet into a micro test tube

20 μl clear supernatant
140 μl buffer mixture (F)
20 μl molybdate (B)
20 μl ascorbic acid (C)

Mix with vibrator and allow to stand at room temperature for 15 minutes. Read absorbance in 10 mm microcuvette at 870 nm (maximum) or any wavelength between 600 and 900 nm against a blank with water instead of serum. Prepare a standard with 10 μl working standard (H) instead of serum. If a larger series is processed, the analysis may be interrupted after the addition of buffer mixture (F) to the supernatant (pH brought to 4–4.1).

Calculation

$$\frac{A_{\text{sample}}}{A_{\text{standard}}} \times \text{standard (mg/100 ml)} = \text{mg P/100 ml serum}$$

With $P < 3$ mg/100 ml it is suggested that the amount of serum and reagents be doubled and that a 20-mm microcuvette be used for measurement.

Normal serum values: 2–5 mg P/100 ml.

PROTEIN

Method 1: determination with the biuret reaction

Literature: Henry, R. J., C. Sobel, and S. Berkman, Anal. Chem. **29**, 1491 (1957).

Principle

Proteins form a colored complex with copper ions in alkaline solutions (biuret complex). The concentration of the color complex is determined photometrically.

Reagents

A. *Biuret reagent:* a) dissolve 1.73 g $CuSO_4 \times 5\ H_2O$ in about 10 ml hot redistilled water; b) dissolve 17.3 g sodium citrate and 10 g anhydrous sodium carbonate in about 80 ml redistilled water with heating. When cool add (a) to (b) while stirring and dilute to 100 ml. Stored in a brown bottle, the reagent is stable indefinitely.
B. *NaOH* 3% in redistilled water
C. *Protein standard:* a clear serum may be used; determine total protein with Kjeldahl analysis and correct for nonprotein nitrogen. A solution of bovine serum albumin or a commercial standard serum may be used alternatively. Saturated with benzoic acid and stored in the refrigerator, protein standard solutions are stable for several months.

Procedure

Required amount of serum: 5 μl
Pipet into a micro test tube

250 μl NaOH (B)
5 μl serum

Mix with vibrator and immediately add

50 μl biuret reagent (A)

Mix and allow to stand at room temperature for at least 15 minutes. Prepare a blank with 5 μl H_2O and a standard with 5 μl protein standard instead of serum. Read absorbance in 10-mm microcuvettes against a blank at 530–580 nm. The color is stable for several hours. If the assay mixture with serum is turbid (lipemic serum), add about 150 μl ether, mix with vibrator for 30 seconds, centrifuge and remove ether phase. Read the absorbance in the now clear solution.

Calculation

$$\frac{A_{sample}}{A_{standard}} \times \text{concentration of standard (g/100 ml)} = \text{g protein/100 ml}$$

Normal values: 6.5–8 g protein/100 ml serum.

Method 2: Determination of copper bound in the biuret reaction

Literature: Mattenheimer, H., Z. Physiol. Chem. **316**, 202 (1959) (micromethod); Nielsen, H., Acta Chem. Scand. **12**, 38 (1958).

Principle

Copper bound by protein in the biuret reaction is determined photometrically as a colored complex with sodium diethyldithiocarbamate. Serum protein is separated from peptides and other copper-binding substances, *e.g.*, glucose, by precipitation with trichloroacetic acid and then redissolved in a sodium phosphate solution. The method is about 50 times more sensitive than the biuret method.

Reagents

A. *Trichloroacetic acid* (TCA) 10%
B. $Na_3PO_4 \times 12\ H_2O$ solution 5%
C. $Na_3PO_4 \times 12\ H_2O$ solution 5% with 0.3% Gum Arabic, heat to boiling and filter.
D. $Cu_3(PO_4)_2$ freshly prepared: add $CuSO_4$ (approximately 4%) dropwise to about 5 ml solution B. Centrifuge and wash $Cu_3(PO_4)_2$ precipitate repeatedly with redistilled water. Prepare fresh every day and use the wet precipitate.
E. *Sodium diethyldithiocarbamate:* use the crystals.
F. *NaCl solution* 0.9%

Procedure

Required amount of serum: 5 μl. Dilute serum to 1:50 with NaCl (F) (from 250 μl NaCl solution remove 5 μl and add 5 μl serum with the same pipet).

Pipet into a micro test tube

20 μl diluted serum
40 μl TCA (A)

Mix with vibrator and centrifuge at high speed. Aspirate off supernatant with a polyethylene pipet with a fine tip (suction pump). Add to the precipitate

100 μl phosphate solution (B)

Add one "flea" (page 24), close with rubber stopper and stir* with device described in Figure 18 until all protein is dissolved. Then add Cu-phosphate (D) with a small stainless steel loop and stir* for 45 minutes. Remove "flea" with a magnet and excess Cu-phosphate by centrifuging (Cu-phosphate must be present in excess). Pipet into a micro test tube (without disturbing the Cu-phosphate precipitate)

40 μl clear supernatant
200 μl phosphate solution (C)
1 crystal (E)

---

240 μl total Cu-assay mixture

Mix with vibrator and read absorbance after 15 minutes at 440 nm or nearby wavelength in a 10-mm microcuvette against a blank.
Blank: to 100 μl phosphate solution (B) add Cu-phosphate (D) and proceed as directed above. The absorbance of the blank read against phosphate solution (B) varies slightly with the Cu-phosphate preparation and depends on the temperature. The blank value should not be higher than 0.150. Total dilution of the serum sample

$$= \frac{1}{50} \times \frac{20}{100} \times \frac{40}{240} = 1:1500$$

Calculation

1) Based on a serum protein standard. Process together a commercial standard serum of known protein concentration and the unknown sample.

* Stirring can also be accomplished by intensive vibration (*e.g.*, Eppendorf microvibrator, page 31). No "flea" needs to be added.

$$\frac{A_{sample}}{A_{standard}} \times \text{standard (g protein/100 ml)} = \text{g protein/100 ml serum}$$

2) Based on a standard curve. Construction of standard curve.
Dilute 1 ml serum 1:50 with NaCl solution (F). To 2 ml diluted serum add 4 ml TCA (A), mix and centrifuge. Decant supernatant and blot up droplets from the glass wall with filter paper. Dissolve precipitate in 10 ml phosphate solution. Determine protein concentration by Kjeldahl analysis. With the remaining solution, prepare serial dilutions with phosphate solution (B). To 100 μl of each dilution add Cu-phosphate (D) and continue as described above. On graph paper plot absorbance over "μg protein per ml Cu-assay mixture" (= 4.17 × μg protein per 240 μl Cu-assay mixture). The relation is linear. To calculate the concentration in a serum sample, read "μg protein per ml Cu-assay mixture" for the measured absorbance on the standard curve and substitute into the following formula

$$\frac{(\mu\text{g protein/ml Cu-assay mixture}) \times \text{dilution of sample}}{10{,}000} = \text{g protein/100 ml serum}$$

Example (based on a published standard curve; ref. H. Mattenheimer):

$$A_{sample} = 0.900 = 51.57\ \mu\text{g protein/ml Cu-assay mixture}$$

Total dilution 1 : 1500

$$\frac{51.57 \times 1500}{10{,}000} = 7.74\ \text{g protein/100 ml serum}$$

The standard curve for serum protein is also valid for spinal fluid. Dilute spinal fluid 1:10 with NaCl. Other protein solutions, *e.g.*, tissue extracts, require separate standard curves because of the different Cu-binding capacity of various proteins.

BLOOD SUGAR (*o*-toluidine method)

Literature: Zender, R., Clin. Chim. Acta **8**, 351 (1963); Hyvärinen, A., and E. A. Nikkila, Clin. Chim. Acta **7**, 140 (1962).

Principle

Glucose forms a fairly specific colored compound with *o*-toluidine in acetic acid. The concentration of the color is determined photometrically.

Reagents

A. *Trichloroacetic acid* (TCA) 3%
B. *o-toluidine reagent:* dissolve 270 mg thiourea and 10 ml *o*-toluidine in 90 ml glacial acetic acid. Store in the dark.
C. *Glucose standard:* dissolve 100.0 mg glucose (dried in desiccator over phosphopentoxide) in saturated benzoic acid solution to 100 ml. The solution is stable indefinitely.

Procedure

Required amount of blood: 10 μl
Pipet into a micro test tube

10 μl blood
100 μl TCA (A)

Mix with vibrator and after a few minutes centrifuge. Pipet into a micro test tube

40 μl supernatant
200 μl reagent (B)

Mix, close test tube with Parafilm and incubate in boiling water for exactly 8 minutes. Cool immediately in cold water. After an additional 10 minutes read absorbance in 10-mm microcuvette at 570–650 nm (maximum at 630 nm) against a blank with 10 μl redistilled water instead of blood. Prepare a standard with 10 μl glucose standard (C) instead of blood.

Calculation

$$\frac{A_{sample}}{A_{standard}} \times 100 = \text{mg glucose/100 ml blood}$$

Remark

Construct one calibration curve with glucose concentrations up to 800 mg/100 ml to verify the linearity of the relationship at the selected wavelength. If deviation from Beer's law is found above a certain concentration, blood samples with correspondingly high glucose content must be diluted.

Normal values: 70–110 mg glucose/100 ml blood

URIC ACID (Colorimetric method)

Literature: Henry, R. J., C. Sobel, and J. Kim, Am. J. Clin, Pathol. **28**, 152, 645 (1957) (micromethod).

Principle

Uric acid reduces phosphotungstate in alkaline solution to a tungsten blue which is determined photometrically.

Reagents

A. *Sodium tungstate solution* 10%: dissolve 10 g $Na_2WO_4 \times 2\,H_2O$ (molybdenum-free) in 100 ml redistilled water.

B. H_2SO_4 0.66N

C. *Phosphotungstic acid reagent:* dissolve 40 g $Na_2WO_4 \times 2\,H_2O$ (molybdenum-free) in about 300 ml redistilled water, add 32 ml 85% phosphoric acid. Reflux gently for 2 hours. Cool to room temperature and dilute to 1000 ml with redistilled water. Dissolve 32 g $Li_2SO_4 \times H_2O$ in reagent. Stable indefinitely in refrigerator.

D. *Sodium carbonate solution* 14% (w/v): dissolve 14 g anhydrous Na_2CO_3 in redistilled water to 100 ml. Store in a polyethylene bottle.

E. *Uric acid standard:* see page 121. Dilute this standard (30 mg uric acid/100 ml) 1:30 with redistilled water. 1 ml = 10 μg uric acid.

Procedure

Required amount of serum: 50 μl

Pipet into a 1-ml centrifuge tube	
	50 μl serum 400 μl redistilled water
Mix with vibrator and add	
	25 μl H_2SO_4 (B) 25 μl Na-tungstate (A)
Mix, allow to stand for a few minutes and centrifuge. Pipet into a micro test tube	
	150 μl supernatant 50 μl Na_2CO_3 (D) 50 μl reagent (C)

Mix with vibrator and allow to stand at room temperature for 15 minutes. Read absorbance within the following 30 minutes in 10-mm microcuvettes at 640–720 nm (maximum at 710 nm) against a blank with 150 μl redistilled water instead of supernatant. Prepare a standard with 150 μl diluted standard solution (E) instead of supernatant. Use the same pipet for supernatant, water and standard.

Calculation

$$\frac{A_{sample}}{A_{standard}} \times F = \text{mg uric acid/100 ml serum}$$

The assay mixture contains $\frac{3}{10}$ = 15 μl of 50 μl serum and the amount of uric acid in the standard assay mixture = 1.5 μg

$$F = 1.5 \times \frac{100}{15} = 10$$

F must be recalculated if different volumes and/or different concentrations of the standard are employed.
Normal serum values:

men	2.7–7 mg/100 ml
women	1.5–6 mg/100 ml

For the enzymatic determination of uric acid see page 121.

MAGNESIUM

Literature: Sky-Peck, H. H., Clin. Chem. **10**, 391 (1964).

Principle

Magnesium ions form a red color complex with Thiazole Yellow. The color intensity is proportional to the Mg^{++}-concentration and is determined photometrically.

Reagents

A. *Trichloroacetic acid* (TCA) 5% (w/v)

B. *Polyvinyl alcohol* (Elvanol, Du Pont) 0.015% (w/v): dissolve reagent by gently warming in a water bath. Thymol crystals may be added as a preservative.

C. *Thiazole Yellow stock solution:* dissolve 35 mg Thiazole Yellow (methylbenzothiazole–[1, 3]–4,4′–diazoaminobenzole–2,2disulfonate–Na_2) in 100 ml B. The reagent is light-sensitive and should be kept in a brown bottle.

D. *Thiazole Yellow working solution:* dilute one part (C) with 9 parts (B).

E. *Lithium hydroxide* 2N: dissolve 8.392 g $LiOH \times H_2O$ per 100 ml redistilled water. Store in a polyethylene bottle.

F. *Magnesium standard,* 5 mg/100 ml: in a 100-ml volumetric flask dissolve 50.67 mg $MgSO_4 \times 7\ H_2O$ in redistilled water and fill to the mark.

Procedure

Required amount of serum: 50 μl
Pipet into a 1 ml test tube

	50 μl serum 450 μl TCA (A)
Mix with vibrator and allow to stand for at least 10 minutes. Centrifuge at high speed. Pipet into a micro test tube	
	200 μl clear supernatant 100 μl Thiazole Yellow (D) 100 μl LiOH (E)

Mix with vibrator and allow to stand for at least 15 minutes at room temperature. The color is stable for several hours. Read absorbance at 520–570 nm in 10-mm microcuvettes against a blank with 50 μl redistilled water instead of serum. Prepare a standard with 50 μl Mg standard (F) instead of serum.

Calculation

$$\frac{A_{\text{sample}}}{A_{\text{standard}}} \times \text{concentration of standard (mg/100 ml)} =$$

$$= \text{mg Mg/100 ml serum}$$

$$(\text{mg Mg/100 ml}) \times 0.86 = \text{meq Mg/liter}$$

If not enough serum is available, deproteinize 25 μl serum with 225 μl TCA.

Normal serum values: 1.6–2.2 mg Mg/100 ml = 1.3–1.8 meq/l

CHLORIDE

Literature: Schales, O., and S. S. Schales, J. Biol. Chem. **140**, 879 (1941); micromodification according to Beckman Technical Bulletin #6072 C.

Principle

Chloride is titrated with mercuric nitrate in acid solution, forming soluble but undissociated mercuric chloride. Excess mercuric ions react with diphenylcarbazone to form a violet color complex. Its appearance indicates the end point.

Reagents

A. *Mercuric nitrate solution,* 0.10N: in a 100-ml volumetric flask dissolve 1.623 g mercuric nitrate in redistilled water, add 1 ml conc. nitric acid and fill to the mark.

B. *Nitric acid* approx. 0.03N: dilute 0.02 ml conc. nitric acid to 100 ml with redistilled water.

C. *Indicator solution:* dissolve 100 mg diphenylcarbazone in 100 ml 95% ethanol. Store the orange-red solution in a dark bottle in the refrigerator.

D. *Chloride standard* 0.1N: in a 100-ml volumetric flask dissolve 0.584 g dried NaCl in redistilled water and fill to the mark.

Procedure

Required amount of serum: 10 μl
Pipet into a microtitrator

10 μl serum
80 μl nitric acid (B)
80 μl indicator (C)

Mix and titrate with mercuric nitrate solution (A) to a definite violet color.

Titrate a standard with 10 μl chloride standard and a blank with 10 μl redistilled water instead of serum. Use the same pipet for serum, standard and water. The Beckman Spinco microtitrator 153 is recommended for the titration (see page 29).

Calculation

$$\frac{\mu l_{\text{sample}} - \mu l_{\text{blank}}}{\mu l_{\text{standard}} - \mu l_{\text{blank}}} \times 100 = \text{meq chloride/liter serum}$$

$$\text{meq chloride/liter} \times 3.55 = \text{mg chloride/100 ml}$$

Normal serum values: 97–108 meq/l = 344–383 mg/100 ml.

CHOLESTEROL

Literature: Watson, D., Clin. Chim. Acta **5**, 637 (1961); Richterich, R., and K. Lauber, Klin. Wochschr. **40**, 1252 (1962) (micromethod).

Principle

In a water-free medium cholesterol reacts with acetic anhydride and conc. sulfuric acid to give a blue-green color complex. "Total cholesterol" is determined by this method. Deproteinization is not required. The assay mixture is freed from water by an excess of acetic anhydride. Protein precipitated by dehydration is dispersed with 2,5-dimethyl-benzoyl-sulfonic acid.

Reagents

A. *Cholesterol reagent:* dissolve 5.6 g 2,5-dimethyl-benzoyl-sulfonic acid × $2H_2O$ acid in 100 ml glacial acetic acid and add 300 ml acetic anhydride and 100 ml glacial acetic acid. The reagent is stable for one year in a tightly closed bottle.

B. *Cholesterol standard,* 400 mg/100 ml: in a 100-ml volumetric flask dissolve 400 mg purified cholesterol in about 90 ml glacial acetic acid with gentle warming, allow to cool and fill to 100 ml with glacial acetic acid.

C. *Conc. H_2SO_4*

Procedure

All glassware must be dry.
Required amount of serum: 10 μl, free of visible hemolysis.
Pipet into a 1-ml test tube

	10 μl serum
	250 μl reagent (A)
Mix with vibrator and allow to stand for 5 minutes in a water bath of room temperature. Hold test tube horizontally and place on the wall	
	50 μl H_2SO_4 (C)

Mix in H_2SO_4 with vibrator. Allow to stand for 10 minutes in room temperature water bath. Read absorbance 10–15 minutes after mixing with H_2SO_4 in a 10-mm microcuvette at 560–580 nm against a blank. Prepare a blank with 10 μl redistilled water and a standard with 10 μl cholesterol standard (B) instead of serum. Use the same pipet for serum, standard and water.

Calculation

$$\frac{A_{sample}}{A_{standard}} \times 400 = \text{mg total cholesterol/100 ml serum}$$

Normal values: 120–250 mg/100 ml serum.

HEMOGLOBIN

Literature: Hainline, A., Standard Methods of Clinical Chemistry **2**, 49 (1958).

Principle

In a potassium ferricyanide–potassium cyanide solution, hemoglobin is oxidized to methemoglobin and converted into cyanmethemoglobin, which is determined photometrically at 540 nm.

Reagent

Potassium ferricyanide–cyanide solution: dissolve 5 mg KCN, 20 mg $K_3Fe(CN)_6$ and 100 mg $NaHCO_3$ in 100 ml redistilled water. Stored in a brown bottle and in the absence of direct light, the solution is stable for about one month.

Procedure

Required amount of blood: 10 μl, *e.g.*, collect capillary blood directly with a 10-μl constriction pipet. If venous blood is drawn, an anticoagulant must be added.

Pipet into a test tube or directly into a 10-mm macrocuvette	2.5 ml reagent
	10 μl blood

(Rinse blood into the reagent.)
Allow to stand for at least 20 minutes. Read absorbance against reagent as blank at 540 nm.

Calculation

The calculation is based on the molar extinction coefficient $\varepsilon = 11.0 \times 10^3$ (Clin. Chim. Acta **5**, 719 [1960]) and the molecular weight of hemoglobin (monomer) = 16,114.

$$\frac{A_{sample} \times 16{,}114}{11.0 \times 10^3} \times 0.1 \times \frac{2.510}{0.010} = A_{sample} \times 36.8 = \text{g Hb/100 ml blood}$$

When measurements are made at a different wavelength, a certified commercial cyanmethemoglobin standard must be used.
Normal blood values:

men	16–18 g Hb/100 ml
women	14–16 g Hb/100 ml

INULIN (Renal function test)

Literature: Führ, J., J. Kaczmarczyk, and C. D. Krüttgen, Klin. Wochschr. **33**, 729 (1955); Führ, J., Ärztl. Labor **4**, 79 (1958) (micromethod).

Principle

Inulin reacts with anthrone to form a blue-green compound which is determined photometrically.

Reagents

A. *Zinc sulfate solution* 10%: dissolve 5 g $ZnSO_4 \times 7\ H_2O$ to 50 ml with redistilled water.
B. *NaOH* 0.5N
C. *Anthrone reagent:* add 125 ml conc. H_2SO_4 (D = 1.84) slowly while stirring and cooling (caution!) to 50 ml redistilled water. Dissolve 200 mg anthrone in 100 ml of the diluted acid. The anthrone reagent is stable for only a few days.
D. *Inulin standard,* 50 mg/100 ml: in a 100-ml volumetric flask dissolve 50 mg dry inulin in redistilled water and fill to the mark.

Procedure

Required amount of serum: 25 μl (capillary blood may be used).

Pipet into a micro test tube	100 μl redistilled water 50 μl $ZnSO_4$ (A) 50 μl NaOH (B)
Mix with vibrator, then add	25 μl serum
Mix, allow to stand for 2 minutes and centrifuge. Pipet into a micro test tube	250 μl anthrone reagent (C) ice cold 25 μl supernatant

Mix with vibrator and incubate for exactly 10 minutes in a water bath or on a heating block at 55°C. Place test tubes in an ice bath until measurements are made. Read absorbance in 10-mm microcuvettes at 550–600 nm against a blank. Prepare a blank with 25 μl redistilled water and a standard with 25 μl (D) instead of serum. Use the same pipet for serum, standard and water.

Calculation

$$\frac{A_{\text{sample}}}{A_{\text{standard}}} \times 50 = \text{mg inulin/100 ml serum}$$

If para-aminohippuric acid is to be determined at the same time, double the amount of H_2O, $ZnSO_4$, NaOH and serum.

p-AMINOHIPPURIC ACID (PAH) (Renal function test)

Literature: Führ, J., J. Kaczmarczyk, and C. D. Krüttgen, Klin. Wochschr. **33**, 729 (1955); Führ, J., Ärztl. Labor **4**, 79 (1958) (micromethod).

Principle

PAH is converted into a red diazo dye which is determined photometrically.

Reagents

A. *Zinc sulfate* 10%: dissolve 5 g $ZnSO_4 \times 7\ H_2O$ to 50 ml with redistilled water.

B. *NaOH* 0.5N

C. *HCl* 0.1N

D. *Sodium nitrite* 0.1%: dissolve 10 mg $NaNO_2$ in 10 ml redistilled water. Solution is unstable, prepare fresh every day.

E. *Amidosulfonic acid* 0.5%: dissolve 250 mg amidosulfonic acid in 50 ml redistilled water. Stored in the refrigerator, the solution is stable for about three weeks.

F. *Ethyl-α-naphtylaminedihydrobromide* 0.1%: dissolve 100 mg substance in 10 ml warm methanol and dilute to 100 ml with redistilled water. If the dihydrobromide is not available, dissolve 100 mg ethyl-α-naphthylamine and add 2–3 drops 10% HBr.

G. *PAH standard,* 2 mg/100 ml: dissolve 20 mg PAH in 100 ml redistilled water. For working standard dilute 1:10 with water = 2 mg/100 ml.

Procedure

Required amount of serum: 25 μl (capillary blood may be used).
Pipet into a micro test tube

100 μl redistilled water
50 μl $ZnSO_4$ (A)
50 μl NaOH (B)

Mix with vibrator, then add

25 μl serum

Mix, allow to stand for 2 minutes and centrifuge. Pipet into a micro test tube

200 μl supernatant
50 μl HCl (C)
20 μl $NaNO_2$ (D)

Mix and after 5 minutes add

20 μl amidosulfonic acid (E)

Mix and after 5 minutes add

20 μl ethyl-α-naphthylamine (F)

Mix with vibrator. The color development is very slow and is completed after about two hours. Read absorbance in 10-mm microcuvettes at 550 nm (or nearby wavelength) against a blank. Prepare a blank with 25 μl redistilled water and a standard with 25 μl inulin standard instead of serum.

Calculation

$$\frac{A_{sample}}{A_{standard}} \times 2 = \text{mg PAH/100 ml serum}$$

If inulin is to be determined at the same time, double the amount of H_2O, $ZnSO_4$, NaOH and serum.

SODIUM, POTASSIUM AND CALCIUM (Flame photometry)

Literature: Stamm, D., and R. Herrmann, Z. Klin. Chem. **3**, 193 (1965) (micromethod).

The authors adapted a conventional milliliter method for the flame photometric analysis of Na, K and Ca in a single 15-μl sample of serum, and suggested the use of the Eppendorf Microliter System (page 30) in combination with the Eppendorf flame photometer.

Equipment

Eppendorf microliter pipets: 5, 10, 500 and 1000 μl; reaction vessels; transfer rack; rotary shaker; Eppendorf flame photometer with interference filters 589 nm for Na, 767 nm for K, and 622 nm for Ca.

To reduce to 16–18 seconds the time needed to reach maximum deflection of the galvanometer, the aspiration tubing is shortened to 8 cm; the protective screen, normally attached to the lower end of the tubing to avoid clogging of the atomizer, must be removed.

The following adjustments of the photometer are suggested to achieve a sample flow of 1200 μl per minute:

Element	*Compressed Air** kg/cm^2	1/min.		*Fuel Gas* pressure (mm H_2O)	1/min.	*Multiplier* step	voltage
Sodium	0.5	4	propane	210	0.30	3–4	500–580
Potassium	0.5	4	propane	210	0.30	9	1000
Calcium	0.5	4	acetylene	460–500	0.35	9	1000

* Does not include the protective gas flow around the flame of *ca.* 5 l/min.

Reagents

The reagents are products of E. Merck, Darmstadt, Germany, and are available through Brinkmann Instruments, Westbury, New York.

A. *Calibration solution:* Titrisol # 9976, containing 143.5 meq/l Na, 3.93 meq/l K and 5.05 meq/l Ca.

B. *Diluent:* Titrisol #9975; serves also as blank solution for Na.

C. *Potassium blank*: Titrisol #9977

D. *Calcium blank:* Titrisol #9978
Solutions A–D are concentrates and must be diluted with redistilled water as indicated on the containers.

Procedure

1. Calibration
   To exactly 100 ml of diluent (B) add exactly 1 ml of calibration solution (A). The dilution is 1:101 and is identical to the dilution used for the unknown serum samples.
   Transfer 1.5 ml aliquots into reaction vessels.

   Blank solutions
   Sodium: diluent (B)
   Potassium: 100 ml (B) plus 1 ml potassium blank (C).
   Calcium: 100 ml diluent (B) plus 1 ml calcium blank (D).
   Transfer 1.5 ml aliquots into reaction vessels.
   Zero points and calibration points are adjusted with the respective blanks and the diluted calibration solution. Galvanometer readings are taken after maximally 20 seconds. The calibration should be repeated after about five determinations.

2. Determination in serum.
   Required amount of serum: 2 × 15 μl (for duplicates). Venous blood must be drawn without stasis. If blood is drawn for other analyses at the same time, only the first sample should be used for electrolyte measurements. Serum must be free of visible hemolysis and should be separated from the clot not later than one hour after the blood was drawn.

Pipet into a reaction vessel (500 and 1000 μl pipets)	1500 μl diluent (B)
and add (5 and 10 μl pipets)	15 μl serum
	Dilution of sample 1:101

Close vessels and mix for 3 minutes with the rotary shaker. The samples are now ready for flame photometry. Galvanometer readings must be taken maximally after 20 seconds from the beginning of aspiration.
The calculation is based on the calibration data.

Remark

The atomizer and burner assembly has to be cleaned frequently. Since the protective screen is omitted, fibrin may clog the atomizer. Prolongation of the time to reach maximum galvanometer deflection or fluctuation indicates contamination.

Chapter 5

Enzymatic Determination of Metabolites

ENZYMATIC DETERMINATION OF ADP AND AMP

Literature: Hockerts, T., and W. Lamprecht. Die Medizinische **8,** 289 (1957); Thorn, W., G. Pfleiderer, R. A. Frowein, and G. Ross, Pflügers Arch. Physiol. **261,** 334 (1955).

Principle

ADP and AMP are determined with enzyme reactions that can be coupled with a NADH dependent system.

a) ADP is phosphorylated to ATP with phosphoenol pyruvate (PEP) and pyruvate kinase (PK). Pyruvate formed is reduced with NADH and lactate dehydrogenase (LDH).

$$\text{ADP} + \text{PEP} \underset{}{\overset{\text{PK}}{\rightleftharpoons}} \text{ATP} + \text{pyruvate} \qquad (1)$$

$$\text{pyruvate} + \text{NADH} + \text{H}^+ \underset{}{\overset{\text{LDH}}{\rightleftharpoons}} \text{lactate} + \text{NAD}^+ \qquad (2)$$

The amount of NADH oxidized is equivalent to the concentration of ADP.

b) After completion of reactions (1) and (2), AMP can be determined in the same assay mixture. The amounts of ATP formed in reaction (1) and of ATP present in blood are sufficient to convert AMP into ADP with myokinase (MK).

$$AMP + ATP \xrightleftharpoons{MK} 2\ ADP \qquad (3)$$

ADP then reacts according to reaction (1) and (2). The reagents already contained in the mixture are sufficient for the second ADP assay. Note for the calculation that 2 moles of ADP are formed per mole of AMP.

Reagents

A. *Triethanolamine* (1.0M)-*K_2CO_3* (1.3M): in 100 ml redistilled water dissolve 18.56 g triethanolamine hydrochloride and 17.96 g anhydrous K_2CO_3.

B. *Phosphoenol pyruvate solution* 1×10^{-2}M with *$MgSO_4$* 0.4M and *KCl* 1.3M: in 1 ml redistilled water dissolve 2.08 mg PEP (Na-salt $\times$ H_2O) or 4.65 mg PEP-cyclohexylammonium salt, 98.5 mg $MgSO_4 \times 7\ H_2O$ and 96.9 mg KCl.

C. *Lactate dehydrogenase* (LDH): minimum activity 300 U/mg. Dilute commercial crystalline LDH suspension with 2.2M ammonium sulfate to give 1 mg/ml.

D. *NADH solution* 5×10^{-3}M: dissolve 3.55 mg NADH-Na_2 in 1 ml redistilled water. Note purity of preparation and increase amount if necessary.

E. *Pyruvate kinase* (PK): minimum activity 100 U/mg. Dilute commercial crystalline PK suspension with 2.1M ammonium sulfate to give 1 mg/ml.

F. *Myokinase* (MK): minimum activity 300 U/mg. Dilute commercial MK suspension with 3.2M ammonium sulfate to give 2 mg/ml.

G. *Perchloric acid* 6% (w/v): dilute 5 ml of 70% perchloric acid with redistilled water to make 100 ml.

Procedure

Required amount of blood: 500 μl

It is essential to immediately deproteinize the freshly obtained blood to avoid the breakdown of ATP to ADP.

Pipet into a 1.5 ml test tube

500 μl perchloric acid (G) (ice cold)
500 μl blood

Mix with vibrator and centrifuge.

Pipet into a 1.5 ml test tube

400 μl clear supernatant
100 μl triethanolamine (A)

Mix with vibrator and leave in ice bath for 15 minutes; potassium perchlorate precipitates. Centrifuge and transfer supernatant into another test tube in a water bath of 25°C. The solution is buffered at pH 7.5.

Pipet into a 10-mm microcuvette

200 μl supernatant
15 μl PEP (B)
10 μl NADH (D)
2 μl LDH (C)

Mix with polyethylene stirrer and read absorbance at 366, 340 or 334 nm. Traces of pyruvate in the PEP preparation and pyruvate in blood react with consumption of NADH in the presence of LDH. When no further decrease in absorbance occurs, read absorbance ($= A_1$) and mix in

2 μl PK (E)
____
229 μl total volume (ADP)

Read absorbance at 1 minute intervals until the reaction comes to a standstill ($= A_2$); then mix in

2 μl MK (F)
____
231 μl total volume (AMP)

Read absorbance again at 1 minute intervals. End point of absorbance decrease $= A_3$.

Calculation:

Determine the end points A_2 and A_3 graphically (example see page 40).

$$A_1 - A_2 = \Delta A \text{ for ADP}$$
$$A_2 - A_3 = \Delta A \text{ for AMP}$$

Mol. wt. ADP = 427.2; AMP = 347.2.
Dilution: 1 ml blood = 1.06 g; 500 μl blood = 530 mg
Water content ~80%. $530 \times \frac{80}{100}$ + 500 μl perchloric acid = 924 μl extract. 400 μl extract + 100 μl buffer = 500 μl buffered solution, of which 200 μl are used for the assay.
Measurement at 366 nm:

ADP

$$\frac{\Delta A}{3.3 \times 10^3} \times 229 = \Delta A \times 0.0694 = \mu\text{moles ADP/229 } \mu\text{l}$$

(assay volume)

$$\frac{\Delta A}{3.3 \times 10^3} \times \frac{229}{200} \times \frac{924}{500} \times \frac{500}{400} \times 10^3 = \Delta A \times 0.802$$
$$= \mu\text{moles ADP/1 ml blood}$$

$$\Delta A \times 0.802 \times \frac{427.2}{10} = \Delta A \times 34.24 = \text{mg ADP/100 ml blood.}$$

AMP

$$\frac{\Delta A}{3.3 \times 10^3} \times \frac{231}{200} \times \frac{924}{500} \times \frac{500}{400} \times 10^3 \times 0.5 = \Delta A \times 0.404$$
$$= \mu\text{moles AMP/1 ml blood}$$

$$\frac{\Delta A}{3.3 \times 10^3} \times 231 \times 0.5 = \Delta A \times 0.035 = \mu\text{moles AMP/231 } \mu\text{l}$$

(assay volume)

$$\Delta A \times 0.404 \times \frac{347.2}{10} = \Delta A \times 14.02 = \text{mg AMP/100 ml blood}$$

Measurement at 340 nm: ADP

$\Delta A \times 0.037$ = μmoles ADP/229 μl (assay volume)
$\Delta A \times 0.426$ = μmoles ADP/ml blood
$\Delta A \times 18.22$ = mg ADP/100 ml blood

AMP

$\Delta A \times 0.018 = \mu$moles AMP/231 μl (assay volume)
$\Delta A \times 0.215 = \mu$moles AMP/ml blood
$\Delta A \times 7.46 =$ mg AMP/100 ml blood

Measurement at 334 nm: ADP

$\Delta A \times 0.038 = \mu$moles ADP/229 μl (assay volume)
$\Delta A \times 0.441 = \mu$moles ADP/ml blood
$\Delta A \times 18.84 =$ mg ADP/100 ml blood

AMP

$\Delta A \times 0.019 = \mu$moles AMP/231 μl (assay volume)
$\Delta A \times 0.222 = \mu$moles AMP/ml blood
$\Delta A \times 7.70 =$ mg AMP/100 ml blood

Normal values in blood:

2.1–4.8 mg ADP/100 ml
0.5–1.2 mg AMP/100 ml

With pipet volumes different from those prescribed, the factors must be recalculated (example on page 114).

ENZYMATIC DETERMINATION OF ATP

Literature: Hockerts, T., and W. Lamprecht, Die Medizinische **8**, 289 (1957); Thorn, W., G. Pfleiderer, R. A. Frowein, and G. Ross, Pflügers Arch. Physiol. **261**, 334 (1955).

Principle

ATP is determined with the enzymes phosphoglycerate kinase (PGK) and glyceraldehyde phosphate dehydrogenase (GAPDH). In the presence of ATP and PGK, 3-phosphoglycerate (3-PG) is phosphorylated to 1,3-diphosphoglycerate (1,3 PGP), which in turn is reduced and dephosphorylated to glyceraldehyde-3-phosphate GAP in the presence of NADH and GAPDH.

$$\text{3-PG} + \text{ATP} \xrightleftharpoons{\text{PGK}} \text{1,3-PGP} + \text{ADP}$$

$$\text{1,3-PGP} + \text{NADH} + \text{H}^+ \xrightleftharpoons{\text{GAPDH}} \text{GAP} + \text{NAD}^+ + \text{P}$$

---

overall reaction:

$$\text{3-PG} + \text{ATP} + \text{NADH} + \text{H}^+ \rightleftharpoons \text{GAP} + \text{NAD}^+ + \text{ADP} + \text{P}.$$

The amount of NADH oxidized is equivalent to the concentration of ATP.

Reagents

A. *Triethanolamine buffer* 0.1M, pH 7.6 with *$MgSO_4$* 4×10^{-3}M and *3-PG* 6×10^{-3}M: in 10 ml buffer dissolve 9.85 mg $MgSO_4 \times 7\ H_2O$ and 32.3 mg 3-phosphoglycerate-tricyclohexylammonium salt × × 3 H_2O.

B. *NADH solution* 1.2×10^{-2}M: dissolve 8.5 mg NADH-Na_2 in 1 ml redistilled water.
Note purity of preparation and increase amount if necessary.

C. *Enzyme mixture* GAPDH/PGK: 4 mg GAPDH and 1 mg PGK per ml. Minimum activity 30 U/mg GAPDH, 150 U/mg PGK. Prepare from commercial crystalline suspensions in ammonium sulfate: *e.g.*, GAPDH 10 mg/ml, PGK 10 mg/ml. Mix 0.4 ml GAPDH, 0.1 ml PGK and 0.5 ml 2.5M ammonium sulfate.

D. *Perchloric acid* 6% (w/v): dilute 5 ml of 70% perchloric acid with 95 ml redistilled water.

Procedure

Required amount of blood: 100 μl
Pipet into micro test tube

100 μl perchloric acid (D) (ice cold)
100 μl blood

Mix with vibrator and centrifuge.
Allow to warm to room temperature.
Pipet into a 10-mm microcuvette

240 μl buffer (A)
4 μl NADH (B)
20 μl clear supernatant

Mix with polyethylene stirrer and read absorbance at 366, 340 or 334 nm ($= A_1$). Mix in

4 μl GAPDH/PGK (C)

268 μl total volume

Read absorbance at 1 minute intervals. End point of absorbance decrease $= A_2$.

Calculation

Determine A_2 graphically (see page 40). $A_1 - A_2 = \Delta A$.
Mol. wt. ATP = 507.19
Dilution: 1 ml blood = 1.06 g; 100 μl = 106 mg
Water content ~80%. $106 \times \frac{80}{100} + 100$ μl perchloric acid = 184.8 μl extract; of which 20 μl are used for the assay.

Measurement at 366 nm:

$$\frac{\Delta A}{3.3 \times 10^3} \times 268 = \Delta A \times 0.081 = \mu\text{moles ATP/268 } \mu\text{l (assay volume)}$$

$$\frac{\Delta A}{3.3 \times 10^3} \times \frac{268}{20} \times \frac{184.8}{100} \times 10^3 = \Delta A \times 7.504 = \mu\text{moles ATP/ml blood}$$

$$\Delta A \times 7.504 \times \frac{507.19}{10} = \Delta A \times 380.6 = \text{mg ATP/100 ml blood.}$$

Measurement at 340 nm:

$\Delta A \times 0.043$ = μmoles ATP/268 μl (assay volume)
$\Delta A \times 3.991$ = μmoles ATP/ml blood
$\Delta A \times 202.4$ = mg ATP/100 ml blood.

Measurement at 334 nm:

$\Delta A \times 0.045$ = μmoles ATP/268 μl (assay volume)
$\Delta A \times 4.123$ = μmoles ATP/ml blood
$\Delta A \times 209.1$ = mg ATP/100 ml blood.

Normal values in blood: 12–30 mg/100 ml
With pipet volumes different from those prescribed, the factors must be recalculated (example on page 114).

ENZYMATIC DETERMINATION OF ALCOHOL

Literature: Bücher, T., and H. Radetzki, Klin. Wochschr. **29**, 615 (1951).

Principle

Ethanol is oxidized by alcohol dehydrogenase (ADH) to acetaldehyde

$$\text{ethanol} + NAD^+ \rightleftharpoons \text{acetaldehyde} + NADH + H^+$$

At alkaline pH and by trapping acetaldehyde with semicarbazide, the equilibrium is virtually shifted completely to the right. NAD^+ is reduced in equimolar amounts and the alcohol concentration can be determined by measurement of NADH.

Reagents

A. *Perchloric acid,* 3.4% (w/v): dilute 2.9 ml 70% perchloric acid to 100 ml with redistilled water.

B. *Buffer solution:* in about 20 ml redistilled water dissolve 1.0 g sodium pyrophosphate ($Na_4P_2O_7 \times 10\ H_2O$), 0.25 g semicarbazide hydrochloride* and 50 mg glycine; add 1 ml 2N NaOH and fill to 30 ml with redistilled water, pH ~ 8.6.

C. *NAD solution* 2.2×10^{-2}M: dissolve 15 mg NAD in 1 ml redistilled water. Note purity of preparation and increase amount if necessary.

D. *Alcohol dehydrogenase:* use commercially available crystalline suspension in ammonium sulfate with 30 mg ADH/ml.

Procedure

Required amount of blood (or serum): 10 μl

Pipet into micro test tube

40 μl perchloric acid
10 μl blood

Mix with vibrator and centrifuge.

Pipet into a 10-mm microcuvette

240 μl buffer (B)
5 μl NAD (C)
5 μl clear supernatant
1 μl ADH (D)

* Semicarbazide often contains traces of ethanol which can be removed by recrystallization from hot water.

Mix with polyethylene stirrer, cap cuvette with Parafilm and incubate for 60 minutes at room temperature. Read absorbance at 366 or 340 nm in 10-mm microcuvettes against a blank which contains water instead of supernatant.

Calculation

The alcohol concentration is read from a standard curve best constructed with glycine ethylester. Dissolve 0.303 g glycine ethylester hydrochloride (mol. wt. 139.5) in 100 ml 0.1N NaOH. After 20 minutes at room temperature the ester is hydrolyzed, and the solution contains exactly 1 g ethanol per liter ($1^0/_{00}$).

Prepare dilutions of $1^0/_{00}$, $0.75^0/_{00}$, $0.25^0/_{00}$ and use 5 μl for analysis in assay mixture instead of supernatant. Plot absorbance over $^0/_{00}$ alcohol. After deproteinization of 10 μl blood only $\frac{1}{10}$ (= 1 μl) are analyzed; it then follows that $1^0/_{00}$ standard = $10^0/_{00}$ alcohol in undiluted blood.

ENZYMATIC DETERMINATION OF BLOOD GLUCOSE

Method 1: with glucose oxidase and peroxidase

Literature: Huggett, A. St. G., and D.A. Nixon, Lancet 1957, Vol. II, 368; Richterich, R., and J.P. Colombo, Klin. Wochschr. **40**, 1208 (1962) (micromethod).

Principle

Glucose-oxidase (GOD) catalyzes the reaction

$$\beta\text{-D-glucose} + H_2O + O_2 \xrightarrow{\text{GOD}} \text{gluconate} + H_2O_2$$

H_2O_2 is generated in equimolar amounts and oxidizes the hydrogen donor *o*-dianisidine (DH_2) in a coupled "indicator reaction" with peroxidase (POD) to a brownish compound (D).

$$H_2O_2 + DH_2 \xrightarrow{\text{POD}} 2\ H_2O + D$$

The concentration of glucose can be determined by colorimetric measurement of the dye. By lowering the pH below 0.5 at the end of the incubation, the color changes to red. The red dye not only has a higher absorbance but also is stable for many hours.

Reagents

A. *Buffer-enzyme mixture:* dissolve 800 µg peroxidase and 5 mg glucose oxidase in 20 ml phosphate buffer 0.12M, pH 7.0.

B. *Chromogen solution:* dissolve 5 mg *o*-dianisidine hydrochloride in 1 ml redistilled water.

C. *Glucose reagent:* with vigorous stirring add 1 part (B) to 100 parts (A). Keep reagent in brown bottle and prepare fresh daily.

D. *Uranyl acetate solution:* dissolve 160 mg uranyl acetate and 900 mg NaCl in 100 ml redistilled water. (Perchloric acid 0.34M may be used for deproteinization instead of uranyl acetate.)

E. *Glucose standard:* 91 µg/ml. Dry glucose over P_2O_5 overnight and dissolve 9.1 mg per 100 ml benzoic acid solution, saturated at room temperature. The solution is stable at room temperature for about one year. Glucose solution must not be used during the first two hours after preparation because GOD oxidizes β-D-glucose faster than the α-isomer. The concentration of the standard solution takes into account the dilution of blood by deproteinization.

F. *Sulfuric acid: ca.* 25%

Procedure

Required amount of blood: 5 μl. Blood can be obtained from the earlobe or the fingertip with a 5-μl constriction pipet.

Pipet into a micro test tube	
	50 μl uranyl acetate (D)
	5 μl blood (rinse pipet)
Mix with vibrator and centrifuge.	
Pipet into a 1-ml test tube	
	10 μl supernatant
	250 μl glucose reagent (C)
Mix and incubate for 40 minutes at room temperature or 20 minutes at 37°C; then add	
	250 μl H_2SO_4 (F)

Immediately mix with vibrator. Read at 500–550 nm in a 10-mm microcuvette against a blank with 10 μl H_2O instead of supernatant. Prepare a standard with 10 μl glucose standard (E) instead of supernatant. Use the same pipet for supernatant, glucose standard and H_2O. No deproteinization is necessary to determine glucose in serum. Dilute 5 μl serum with 50 μl H_2O and use 10 μl of the dilution instead of supernatant.

Calculation

$$\frac{A_{sample}}{A_{standard}} \times 100 = \text{mg glucose/100 ml blood}$$

With concentrations higher than 350 mg/100 ml, repeat determination with 5 μl supernatant + 5 μl H_2O.

Normal values:

50–95 mg/100 ml blood
75–105 mg/100 ml serum

Remarks

It is essential to use glucose oxidase of highest purity. Less pure preparations may contain catalase which decomposes H_2O_2.

Method 2: UV-test

Literature: Slein, M. W., G. T. Cori, and C. F. Cori, J. Biol. Chem. **186**, 763 (1950). Schmidt, F. H., Klin. Wochschr. **39**, 1244 (1961).

Principle

Glucose is phosphorylated to glucose-6-phosphate (glucose-6-ph) by hexokinase (HK) and ATP.

$$\text{glucose} + \text{ATP} \xrightarrow{(\text{HK})} \text{glucose-6-phosphate} + \text{ADP}$$

Glucose-6-ph is oxidized to 6-phosphogluconolactone with glucose-6-ph dehydrogenase (G-6-PDH) and NADP ("indicator reaction").

$$\text{Glucose-6-ph} + \text{NADP}^+ \xrightarrow{(\text{G-6-PDH})} \text{6-phosphogluconolactone} + \text{NADP} + \text{H}^+$$

Glucose is determined by measuring NADPH which is generated in equimolar amounts.

Reagents

A. *Triethanolamine buffer* 0.3M, pH 7.5, with 4×10^{-3}M $MgSO_4$: in 10 ml buffer dissolve 9.9 mg $MgSO_4 \times 7\ H_2O$.

B. *NADP solution* 1.2×10^{-2}M: dissolve 9.2 mg NADP-NaH_2 in 1 ml redistilled water. Note purity of preparation and increase amount if necessary.

C. *ATP-solution* 1.6×10^{-2}M: dissolve 9.7 mg ATP-$Na_2H_2 \times 3\ H_2O$ in 1 ml redistilled water.

D. *Hexokinase/glucose-6-ph dehydrogenase:* 1 mg HK and 2 mg G-6-PDH per ml 3M ammonium sulfate solution pH 7.

E. *Perchloric acid:* with redistilled water dilute 2.85 ml perchloric acid 70% to 100 ml.

Procedure

Required amount of blood: 10 μl. Blood can be obtained from the earlobe or the fingertip with a 10-μl constriction pipet.
Pipet into a micro test tube

100 μl perchloric acid (E)
10 μl blood (rinse pipet)

Mix with vibrator and centrifuge.
Pipet into a 10-mm microcuvette

260 μl buffer (A)
20 μl supernatant
10 μl NADP (B)
10 μl ATP (C)

Mix with polyethylene stirrer and read absorbance at 366, 340 or 334 nm. Mix in

2 μl HK/G-6-PDH (D)

---

302 μl total volume.

Mix with polyethylene stirrer and read absorbance after 10 minutes at 1 minute intervals for 4–5 minutes. Obtain difference in absorbance (ΔA) graphically: see example on page 40.
When ΔA exceeds 0.150, repeat with 10 μl or less supernatant; adjust volume in assay mixture with H_2O; multiply result accordingly.

Calculation

Mol. wt. glucose = 180.15
Dilution: 1 ml blood = 1.06 g; 10 μl = 10.6 mg.
Water content ~ 80%. $10.6 \times \frac{80}{100} + 100$ μl perchloric acid = 108.5 μl extract, of which 20 μl are used for the assay.

Measurement at 366 nm:

$$\frac{\Delta A}{3.3 \times 10^3} \times 302 = \Delta A \times 0.0915 = \mu\text{moles glucose/302 } \mu\text{l}$$

(assay volume)

$$\frac{\Delta A}{3.3 \times 10^3} \times \frac{302}{20} \times \frac{108.5}{10} \times 10^3 = \Delta A \times 49.64$$

$$= \mu\text{moles glucose/ml blood}$$

$$\Delta A \times 49.64 \times \frac{180.15}{10} = \Delta A \times 894.3 = \text{mg glucose/100 ml blood.}$$

Measurement at 340 nm:

ΔA × 0.0486 = μmoles glucose/302 μl (assay volume)
ΔA × 26.40 = μmoles glucose/ml blood
ΔA × 475.7 = mg glucose/100 ml blood

Measurement at 334 nm:

$\Delta A \times 0.0502 = \mu$moles glucose/302 μl (assay volume)
$\Delta A \times 27.27 = \mu$moles glucose/ml blood
$\Delta A \times 491.3 =$ mg glucose/100 ml blood

With pipet volumes different from those prescribed, the factors must be recalculated (example on page 114).

Normal values: 45–95 mg glucose/100 mg blood.

ENZYMATIC DETERMINATION OF PYRUVATE

Literature: Hess, B., Klin. Wochschr. **33**, 540 (1955); Thorn, W., G. Pfleiderer, R. A. Frowein, and G. Ross, Pflügers Arch. Physiol. **261**, 334 (1955).

Principle

Pyruvate is reduced to lactate by lactate dehydrogenase (LDH) and NADH

$$\text{Pyruvate} + \text{NADH} + \text{H}^+ \xrightleftharpoons{\text{LDH}} \text{lactate} + \text{NAD}^+$$

The reduction is complete at pH 6.8 and excess of NADH. The concentration of pyruvate is determined by measuring the decrease of NADH which is oxidized in equimolar amounts.

Reagents

A. *Phosphate solution,* 1.1 M: dissolve 1.916 g K_2HPO_4 in 10 ml redistilled water.

B. *NADH solution* 5×10^{-3}M: dissolve 3.55 mg NADH-Na_2 in 1 ml redistilled water. Note purity of preparation and increase amount if necessary.

C. *Lactate dehydrogenase* (LDH): minimum activity 300 U/mg. Dilute commercial crystalline suspension to 0.75 mg/ml with 2.2 M ammonium sulfate.

D. *Perchloric acid* 6%: dilute 5 ml perchloric acid 70% to 100 ml with redistilled water.

Procedure

Required amount of blood (or serum): 300 µl. To obtain reproducible results blood must be withdrawn without venous stasis.

Pipet into 1-ml test tube

	300 µl blood (or serum)
	300 µl perchloric acid (D)
Mix with vibrator and centrifuge after 5 minutes. Pipet into micro test tube	
	200 µl clear supernatant
	70 µl phosphate (A)

Mix and keep in ice bath for 10 minutes; perchlorate precipitates. Centrifuge and transfer supernatant into another test tube. Allow to warm to room temperature; the pH is now 6.8. Pipet into 10-mm microcuvette

200 μl buffered supernatant
5 μl NADH (B)

Mix with polyethylene stirrer and read absorbance at 366, 340 or 334 nm. Then add

5 μl LDH (C)

210 μl total volume

Mix with polyethylene stirrer and read absorbance at 1 minute intervals for 5 minutes. Obtain difference in absorbance (ΔA) graphically. See example page 40.

Calculation

Mol. wt. of pyruvate = 88.06 (as free acid)
Dilution: 1 ml blood = 1.06 g; 300 μl = 318 mg
Water content ~80%. $318 \times \frac{80}{100} + 300$ μl perchloric acid = 554.4 μl extract. 200 μl extract + 70 μl phosphate = 270 μl buffered solution, of which 200 μl are used for the assay.

Measurement at 366 nm:

$$\frac{\Delta A}{3.3 \times 10^3} \times 210 = \Delta A \times 0.0636 = \mu\text{moles pyruvate/210 } \mu\text{l (assay volume)}$$

$$\frac{\Delta A}{3.3 \times 10^3} \times \frac{210}{200} \times \frac{554.4}{300} \times \frac{270}{200} \times 10^3 = \Delta A \times 0.794 = \mu\text{moles pyruvate/ml blood}$$

$$\Delta A \times 0.794 \times \frac{88.06}{10} = \Delta A \times 6.99 = \text{mg pyruvate/100 ml blood.}$$

Measurement at 340 nm:

ΔA $\times$ 0.0338 = μmoles pyruvate/210 μl (assay volume)
ΔA $\times$ 0.422 = μmoles pyruvate/ml blood
ΔA $\times$ 3.72 = mg pyruvate/100 ml blood.

Measurement at 334 nm:

$\Delta A \times 0.0349 = \mu$moles pyruvate/210 μl (assay volume)
$\Delta A \times 0.436 = \mu$moles pyruvate/ml blood
$\Delta A \times 3.84 =$ mg pyruvate/100 ml blood

Normal values in blood: 0.4–0.6 mg/100 ml

With pipet volumes different from those prescribed, the factors must be recalculated.

Example

Pipet volumes (μl) prescribed	used	*Solution to be pipetted*
300	293	blood and perchloric acid
200	190	supernatants and buffered extract
70	70	phosphate
5	4	NADH
5	4	LDH

The total assay volume becomes 198 μl (instead of 210 μl).
293 μl blood = 310.6 mg. $310.6 \times \frac{80}{100} + 293$ μl = 541.5 μl extract, 190 μl extract + 70 μl phosphate = 260 μl buffered solution, of which 190 μl are used for the assay.
Measurement at 366 nm:

$$\frac{\Delta A}{3.3 \times 10^3} \times 198 = \Delta A \times 0.060 = \mu\text{moles pyruvate/198 } \mu\text{l (assay volume)}$$

$$\frac{\Delta A}{3.3 \times 10^3} \times \frac{198}{190} \times \frac{541.5}{293} \times \frac{260}{190} \times 10^3 = \Delta A \times 0.799\ \mu\text{moles pyruvate/ml blood}$$

$$\Delta A \times 0.799 \times \frac{88.06}{10} = \Delta A \times 7.04 = \text{mg pyruvate/100 ml blood.}$$

ENZYMATIC DETERMINATION OF 2-OXOGLUTARATE
(α-ketoglutarate)

Literature: Beisenherz, G., H. J. Boltze, T. Bücher, R. Czok, K. H. Garbade, E. Meyer-Arendt, and G. Pfleiderer, Z. Naturforsch. **8b**, 555 (1953).

Principle

2-Oxoglutarate is converted into glutamate by glutamate dehydrogenase (GLDH) in the presence of NH_4^+ and NADH

$$\text{2-oxoglutarate} + NADH + H^+ + NH_4^+ \rightleftharpoons \text{glutamate} + NAD^+ + H_2O$$

With an excess of NH_4^+ and NADH, the conversion is quantitative. NADH is oxidized in equimolar quantities and the decrease in absorbance is a measure for the concentration of 2-oxoglutarate.

Reagents

A. *Potassium phosphate solution* 1.0M: dissolve 21.2 g anhydrous K_3PO_4 in redistilled water and dilute to 100 ml.

B. *NADH solution* 8×10^{-3}M: dissolve 5.7 mg NADH-Na_2 in 1 ml phosphate buffer pH 7.6. Note purity of sample and increase amount if necessary.

C. *Glutamate dehydrogenase* (GLDH): 2 mg/ml in 2.8M ammonium sulfate solution (contains sufficient NH_4^+-ions for the reaction).

D. *Perchloric acid* 6%: with redistilled water dilute 5 ml perchloric acid 70% to 100 ml.

Procedure

Required amount of blood (or serum): 500 μl. To obtain reproducible results blood must be drawn without venous stasis.

Pipet into a 1.5-ml test tube

500 μl blood
500 μl perchloric acid (D)

Mix with vibrator and centrifuge.
Pipet into test tube

400 μl clear supernatant
80 μl phosphate (A)

Mix and keep in ice bath for

10 minutes. Perchlorate precipitates. Centrifuge and transfer supernatant into another test tube. Allow to warm to room temperature. The solution is buffered to pH ∿ 7.6. Pipet into a 20-mm microcuvette

375 μl buffered supernatant
5 μl NADH (B)

Mix with polyethylene stirrer and read absorbance at 366, 340 or 334 nm, then add

5 μl GLDH (C)

385 μl total volume

Mix with polyethylene stirrer and read absorbance at 1 minute intervals for 5 minutes. Obtain absorbance difference (ΔA) graphically. See example page 40.

Calculation

Mol. wt. 2-oxoglutarate = 146.10 (as free acid)
Dilution: 1 ml blood = 1.06 g; 500 μl = 530 mg
Water content ~80%. $530 \times \frac{80}{100} + 500$ μl perchloric acid = 924 μl extract, 400 μl extract + 80 μl phosphate = 480 μl buffered extract, of which 375 μl are used for the assay.

Measurement at 366 nm:

$$\frac{\Delta A}{3.3 \times 10^3} \times 385 \times 0.5 = \Delta A \times 0.0583 =$$

μmoles 2-oxoglutarate/385 μl (assay volume)

$$\frac{\Delta A}{3.3 \times 10^3} \times \frac{385}{375} \times \frac{480}{400} \times \frac{924}{500} \times 10^3 \times 0.5 = \Delta A \times 0.345 =$$

μmoles 2-oxoglutarate/ml blood

$$\Delta A \times 0.345 \times \frac{146.10}{10} = \Delta A \times 5.04 \text{ mg 2-oxoglutarate/100 ml blood.}$$

Measurement at 340 nm:

$\Delta A \times 0.031$ = μmoles 2-oxoglutarate/385 μl (assay volume)
$\Delta A \times 0.184$ = μmoles 2-oxoglutarate/ml blood
$\Delta A \times 2.68$ = mg 2-oxoglutarate/100 ml blood.

Measurement at 334 nm:

$\Delta A \times 0.032$ = μmoles 2-oxoglutarate/385 μl (assay volume)
$\Delta A \times 0.190$ = μmoles 2-oxoglutarate/ml blood
$\Delta A \times 2.77$ = mg 2-oxoglutarate/100 ml blood.

With pipet volumes different from those prescribed, the factors must be recalculated (example on page 114).

Normal values in blood: 0.1–0.2 mg/100 ml

ENZYMATIC DETERMINATION OF LACTATE

Literature: Pfleiderer, G., and K. Dose, Biochem. Z. **326**, 436 (1955); Horn, H. D., and H. F. Bruns, Biochim. Biophys. Acta **21**, 378 (1956); Scholz, R., H. Schmitz, T. Bücher, and J. O. Lampen, Biochem. Z. **331**, 71, (1959).

Principle

Lactate is oxidized to pyruvate by lactate dehydrogenase and NAD.

$$\text{Lactate} + \text{NAD}^+ \rightleftharpoons \text{pyruvate} + \text{NADH} + \text{H}^+$$

The equilibrium at neutral pH is far to the side of lactate, but at an alkaline pH, excess NAD, and by trapping of pyruvate with hydrazine the oxidation of lactate is complete. The lactate concentration is determined by measuring the equimolar formation of NADH.

Reagents

A. *Glycine buffer* 0.5M, pH 9, with *hydrazine* 0.4M: in about 8 ml redistilled water dissolve 375 mg glycine and 200 mg hydrazine hydrate (or 520 mg hydrazine sulfate), adjust to pH 9 with NaOH or HCl, and dilute with water to 10 ml.

B. *NAD solution* 2.7×10^{-2}M: dissolve 18 mg NAD in 1 ml redistilled water. Note purity of the sample and increase amount if necessary.

C. *Lactate dehydrogenase* (LDH): minimum activity 300 U/mg. With 2.2M ammonium sulfate dilute commercial crystalline suspension to 1 mg/ml.

D. *Perchloric acid* 6% (w/v): with redistilled water dilute 5 ml perchloric acid 70% to 100 ml.

Procedure

Required amount of blood: 20 μl. To obtain reproducible results blood must be drawn without venous stasis.
Pipet into a micro test tube

20 μl blood
20 μl perchloric acid (D)

Mix with vibrator and centrifuge
after 5 minutes. Dilute supernatant

1 : 1 with redistilled water.

Pipet into a micro test tube

200 μl buffer	(A)
20 μl NAD	(B)
20 μl diluted supernatant	
3 μl LDH	(C)
243 μl total volume	

Mix with vibrator and incubate for 1 hour at 25°C. Transfer into a 10-mm microcuvette and read absorbance against a blank which contains 20 μl perchloric acid diluted 1 + 3 with redistilled water. (Blank should contain the latter instead of diluted supernatant.)

Calculation

Mol. wt. of lactate = 90.08 (as free acid)
Dilution: 1 ml blood = 1.06 g; 20 μl = 21.2 mg.
Water content ~80%. $21.2 \times \frac{80}{100} + 20$ μl perchloric acid = 36.96 μl extract which is further diluted 1 + 1 with redistilled water. Of this dilution 20 μl (= 10 μl extract) are used for the assay.

Measurement at 366 nm:

$$\frac{\Delta A}{3.3 \times 10^3} \times 243 = \Delta A \times 0.0736 = \mu\text{moles lactate}/243\ \mu\text{l}$$

(assay volume)

$$\frac{\Delta A}{3.3 \times 10^3} \times \frac{243}{10} \times \frac{36.96}{20} \times 10^3 = \Delta A \times 13.61$$

$$= \mu\text{moles lactate}/1\ \text{ml blood}$$

$$\Delta A \times 13.61 \times \frac{90.08}{10} = \Delta A \times 122.5 = \text{mg lactate}/100\ \text{ml blood.}$$

Measurement at 340 nm:

$\Delta A \times 0.0391$ = μmoles lactate/243 μl (assay volume)
$\Delta A \times 7.48$ = μmoles lactate/ml blood
$\Delta A \times 65.2$ = mg lactate/100 ml blood.

Measurement at 334 nm:

$\Delta A \times 0.0404$ = μmoles lactate/243 μl (assay volume)
$\Delta A \times 7.48$ = μmoles lactate/ml blood
$\Delta A \times 67.3$ = mg lactate/100 ml blood.

With $\Delta A_{366} > 0.120$ the determination has to be repeated with a more dilute extract, because the relation of ΔA to the concentration of lactate is no longer linear (see Parijs, J., and F. Barbier, Z. Klin. Chem. **3**, 74 [1965]).

With pipet volumes different from those prescribed, the factors must be recalculated (example on page 114).

Normal values in blood: 10–15 mg lactate/100 ml.

ENZYMATIC DETERMINATION OF URIC ACID

Literature: Liddle, L., J. E. Seegmiller, and L. Laster, J. Lab. Clin. Med. **54**, 903 (1959).

Principle

Uric acid absorbs ultraviolet light with a maximum at 292 nm. Uricase catalyzes the oxidation of uric acid to allantoin which does not absorb light at this wavelength. The concentration of uric acid in a sample can be calculated from the absorbance difference before and after treatment with uricase.

Reagents

A. *Glycine buffer stock solution* 0.66M, pH 9.4: dissolve 25 g glycine and 4.4 g NaOH in CO_2-free redistilled water and dilute to 500 ml. Add 3 ml chloroform as a preservative. Store in refrigerator. For use in assay, dilute stock solution 1:10 with CO_2-free redistilled water.
B. *Uricase:* commercial enzyme solutions can be obtained from several manufacturers. Check activity of sample with the calibration procedure. Increase volume in the assay of unknown samples if necessary.
C. *Uric acid standard:* dissolve 30.0 mg purified uric acid (see below) in 10 ml hot redistilled water by addition of 1 ml of a hot saturated solution of lithium carbonate, and dilute to 100 ml with redistilled water. The solution is stable for several months when frozen. A 1:25 dilution is prepared for calibration, 1 ml = 12 μg uric acid.

Procedure

Required amount of serum: 10 μl for assay, 10 μl for serum blank.

Pipet into a 10-mm quartz microcuvette	300 μl diluted buffer (A) 10 μl serum
Mix with polyethylene stirrer and read absorbance at 292 nm against a blank (see below) = $A_{1\ assay}$	
Then add	1 μl uricase (B)

Mix with polyethylene stirrer. The reaction is complete after 20–25 minutes. But to ascertain that the uricase activity is sufficient, a reading

is taken after 5 minutes. At that time ΔA should be more than 30% of the total ΔA. Take final reading after 30 minutes $= A_{2\ assay}$.
Blank: serum contains several substances other than uric acid which absorb at 292 nm. To compensate, a dilution of the uric acid standard is used as a blank. With most sera, the 1:25 diluted standard is adequate, but with some a more or less dilute uric acid solution has to be used. The absorbance of serum against the blank should read 0.4–0.6. To calculate the uric acid concentration in the sample, two additional data are needed.

1) The self-absorption of uricase (enzyme blank). Pipet into microcuvette 310 μl dilute glycine buffer (A) and read absorbance against water $= A_{1\ enzyme}$. Add uricase in an amount equal to that used in test (mostly 1 μl), mix and read absorbance $= A_{2\ enzyme}$.
2) Absorbance change of serum without uricase. A spontaneous change in absorbance at 292 nm occurs under the assay conditions with serum and other biological fluids. To determine the magnitude of this change prepare a serum blank with 300 μl dilute glycine buffer (A) and 10 μl serum. $A_{1\ serum}$ = absorbance directly after addition, $A_{2\ serum}$ = absorbance after 30 minutes incubation.

Calculation

a) $A_{assay} = A_{1\ assay} - A_{2\ assay}$
b) $A_{enzyme} = A_{2\ enzyme} - A_{1\ enzyme}$
c) $A_{serum} = A_{2\ serum} - A_{1\ serum}$

$A_{uric\ acid} = a + b + c$
Molar extinction coefficient of uric acid at 292 nm and pH 9.4 : $\varepsilon = 12.5 \times 10^3$. Mol. wt. of uric acid: 168.12. Total assay volume 311 μl, serum volume 10 μl, 1 cm light path.

$$\frac{A_{uric\ acid}}{12.5 \times 10^3} \times 10^3 \times \frac{168.12}{10} \times \frac{311}{10} = A_{uric\ acid} \times 41.8$$

mg uric acid/100 ml serum

With pipet volumes different from those prescribed, the factor must be recalculated by substituting the volumes actually used into the last quotient of the equation.

Calibration

Calibration is suggested whenever the method is introduced in the laboratory or has not been applied for some time. Calibration is essential to check (1) the purity of the uric acid, (2) the activity of the uricase, and (3) the necessity of making measurements at a different wavelength (between 280 and 300 nm).

Pipet into a 10-mm quartz microcuvette

200 μl dilute buffer (A)
100 μl uric acid standard (12 μg/ml)

Mix with polyethylene stirrer and read absorbance ($= A_1$) at 292 nm against water. Then add

1 μl uricase (B)

Mix and read absorbance at 1 minute intervals. The activity of the enzyme is sufficient if ΔA in the first minute is approximately 0.100. Wait until absorbance does not decrease further (after 3–4 minutes) and read absorbance ($= A_2$).

Calculation of calibration

$$A_{\text{uric acid}} = A_2 - A_1 + A_{\text{enzyme}}$$

With the volumes suggested and a uric acid standard of 12 μg/ml = 1.2 mg/100 ml, $A_{\text{uric acid}}$ should read 0.296.

$$\frac{0.296}{12.5 \times 10^3} \times 10^3 \times \frac{301}{100} \times \frac{168.12}{10} = 1.2 \text{ mg/100 ml}$$

$$\varepsilon_{292} = 12.5 \times 10^3 \text{ (1/mole)}$$

For measurements at a different wavelength (x), ε is calculated from $A_{\text{uric acid}}$ at wavelength x and used in the formula on page 122.

Normal serum values: 2–4 mg/100 ml.

Purification of uric acid

Heat 1 liter redistilled water in a 2-liter Erlenmeyer flask (1). In another flask (2) add 11 g lithium carbonate to 750 ml redistilled water and heat to ~90°C. After most of the salt is dissolved, add 25 g uric acid which dissolves instantly. Filter solution from flask 2 into flask 1. Add 25 ml glacial acetic acid; after 15 minutes add another 40 ml. Let stand for 30 minutes and separate uric acid crystals from the still warm solution by suction filtration. Wash crystals with redistilled water until free of acid. Dry in vacuum. Yield: approximately 23 g.

ENZYMATIC DETERMINATION OF UREA

Literature: Method 1, Standard Methods of Clinical Chemistry **I**, 118 (1953); Method 2, Henry, R. J., Clinical Chemistry (New York: Harper Row, 1964), p. 226.

Principle

Ammonia, released from urea by urease, is determined photometrically with Nessler's reagent (Method 1) or Berthelot's reaction (Method 2).

Method 1: with Nessler's reagent

A. *Phosphate buffer:* dissolve 0.6 g KH_2PO_4 and 2 g Na_2HPO_4 (Sørensen) in redistilled water to 100 ml. Dilute 1 volume with 5.5 volumes redistilled water before use.

B. *Urease solution:* the concentration depends on the activity of the sample and should be such that the urea in the standard solution is 100% hydrolyzed in 5–8 minutes. With Sigma urease Type V, for example, use 20 mg urease per 10 ml redistilled water.

C. *Sodium tungstate solution* 10%: Store in polyethylene bottle.

D. *H_2SO_4* 0.9N: in a volumetric flask dilute 2.5 ml conc. H_2SO_4 with redistilled water to exactly 100 ml. Standardize with 1.00N NaOH (phenolphthalein indicator).

E. *Urea standard:* in a volumetric flask dissolve exactly 42.9 mg urea (dried in desiccator) with redistilled water to 100 ml. 1 ml = 200 μg urea N (= 20 mg/100 ml).

F. *Gum Arabic solution* 1%: boil 1 g Gum Arabic in 100 ml redistilled water and filter.

G. *Nessler's reagent* (a) mercury iodide–potassium iodide (*e.g.*, Fisher)
(b) NaOH, 10% (*e.g.*, Fisher).

Mix 1 part (a) with 5 parts (b) shortly before use. The reagent is stable for only 30 minutes.

Procedure

Required amount of serum: 10 μl
Pipet into a micro test tube

65 μl buffer (A)
10 μl serum
5 μl urease (B)

Mix with vibrator and incubate capped test tube at 37°C for 20 minutes. Then add slowly with frequent mixing	
	10 μl tungstate (C) 10 μl H_2SO_4 (D)
Centrifuge after 10 minutes. Pipet into a micro test tube	
	40 μl clear supernatant 180 μl redistilled water 20 μl Gum Arabic (F) 40 μl Nessler's reagent (G)

Mix and after exactly 10 minutes read absorbance at 400 nm (or nearby wavelength) in a 10-mm microcuvette against a blank containing redistilled water instead of serum. Prepare a urea standard with 10 μl standard solution (E) and treat like serum sample.

Calculation

$$\frac{A_{serum}}{A_{standard}} \times 20 = \text{mg urea-N/100 ml serum}$$

$$\frac{A_{serum}}{A_{standard}} \times 42.9 = \text{mg urea/100 ml serum.}$$

Remark

Turbidity often develops during ammonia analysis with Nessler's reagent, simulating a higher absorption. The danger of turbidity increases with the aging of reagent (a). To avoid turbidity R. Ballentine (Methods in Enzymology Vol. III, p. 992) suggests the following way to prepare Nessler's reagent.

> Prepare an approximate 0.05% methyl cellulose solution in boiling water and filter the hot solution through a coarse porous glass filter. Dilute 1 vol. reagent (a) with 2–5 vol. redistilled water. To 10 ml of the solution add 2.5 ml methyl cellulose solution and 10 ml ice cold 10% NaOH (reagent b). Centrifuge immediately after mixing and filter supernatant through a dry porous glass filter. This solution must be used within 20 minutes. The suggested dilution of reagent (a) with 2–5 parts of water depends on the particular reagent and has to be tested.

Method 2: with Berthelot's reaction, without deproteinization

Reagents

A. *Buffered urease solution:* dissolve 150 mg urease (activity 1000 Sumner units per gram: *e.g.*, Sigma urease Type II) and 1.0 g disodium ethylenediaminetetraacetate in 100 ml redistilled water. Adjust pH to 6.5 with NaOH. The solution is stable for about one month when stored at 4° C.

B. *Phenol-color reagent:* dissolve 50 g phenol and 0.25 g sodium nitroprusside in redistilled water to 1 liter. The solution is stable for about two months when stored in a brown bottle in the dark at 4°C.

C. *Alkali-hypochlorite reagent:* dissolve 25.0 g NaOH and 2.1 g Na-hypochlorite in redistilled water to 1 liter. The solution is stable for about two months when stored in a brown bottle in the dark at 4°C.

D. *Urea standard:* in a volumetric flask dissolve exactly 42.9 mg urea (dried in a desiccator) in redistilled water to 100 ml. 1 ml = 0.2 mg urea N or 0.429 mg urea.

Procedure

Required amount of serum: 10 μl
Pipet into a 5 ml test tube

100 μl urease (A)
10 μl serum

Mix by light swirling and incubate for 15 minutes at 37°C or 30 minutes at 25°C; then add

500 μl phenol reagent (B)
500 μl hypochlorite (C)

Mix with vibrator and incubate for 3 minutes at 50°C or 20 minutes at 37°C or 40 minutes at 25°C. Prepare and treat together with the serum sample: a blank with water instead of serum and a standard with urea standard (D) instead of serum. Use same pipet for serum, standard and water. Add 2 ml redistilled water to samples, blank and standard. Read absorbance at 580 nm (or nearby wavelength) in a 10-mm cuvette against water. With absorbance > 0.8 for the serum sample, dilute an aliquot of the colored solution with redistilled water and multiply absorbance with the dilution factor.

Calculation

$$\frac{A_{serum} - A_{blank}}{A_{standard} - A_{blank}} \times 20 = \text{mg urea N/100 ml serum}$$

$$\text{mg urea-N} \times 2.145 = \text{mg urea}$$

Normal serum values:

8–18 mg urea N/100 ml
17–38 mg urea/100 ml.

Chapter 6

Determination of Enzyme Activity

MALATE DEHYDROGENASE (MDH)

Literature: Bergmeyer, H. U., and E. Bernt, in H. U. Bergmeyer, Methods of Enzymatic Analysis, second printing, revised (New York: Academic Press, 1965), p. 757; Ordell, R., Intern. Congr. Clin. Chem., Stockholm, 1957, summary and abstracts, p. 116.

Principle

Malate dehydrogenase catalyzes the reaction

$$\text{malate} + \text{NAD}^+ \rightleftharpoons \text{oxaloacetate} + \text{NADH} + \text{H}^+$$

Under the experimental conditions the equilibrium is far to the side of NAD and malate. NADH is oxidized in equimolar quantity and the rate of oxidation is a measure for the MDH activity.

Oxaloacetate is unstable in aqueous solutions, being partly decarboxylated to pyruvate. To overcome this difficulty oxaloacetate can be generated in the assay mixture from 2-oxoglutarate and aspartate by glutamate oxaloacetate transaminase (GOT).

$$\text{2-oxoglutarate} + \text{aspartate} \xrightleftharpoons{\text{(GOT)}} \text{glutamate} + \text{oxaloacetate}$$

Reagents

A. *Phosphate buffer* 0.1M, pH 7.5 with *Na-*L*-aspartate* 4.2×10^{-2}M: dissolve 72.7 mg Na-L-aspartate ($\times$ H_2O) in 10 ml phosphate buffer.

B. *2-Oxoglutarate solution* 6×10^{-2}M: dissolve 17 mg Na-2-oxoglutarate in 1.5 ml redistilled water, or 13 mg 2-oxoglutaric acid in *ca.* 1 ml redistilled water, neutralize with *ca.* 0.2 ml 0.1N NaOH and dilute to 1.5 ml with redistilled water.

C. *NADH solution* 1.2×10^{-2}M: dissolve 8.5 mg NADH-Na_2 in 1.0 ml of phosphate buffer, pH 7.5. Observe the purity indicated on the package and increase the amount of NADH-Na_2 if necessary.

D. *Glutamate oxaloacetate transaminase* (GOT): use a commercial suspension with 1 mg enzyme protein per 1 ml 3M ammonium sulfate solution. If necessary dilute with ammonium sulfate solution.

Procedure

Required amount of serum: 10 μl, fresh and free from visible hemolysis.
Wavelength: 366, 340 or 334 nm; incubation temperature: 25°C.
Pipet into a 10-mm microcuvette

	275 μl buffered aspartate (A) 5 μl 2-oxoglutarate (B) 5 μl NADH (C) 5 μl GOT (D)
Mix with polyethylene stirrer and wait for 5 minutes, until the amount of aspartate equivalent to the amount 2-oxoglutarate is converted into oxaloacetate. Then mix in	
	10 μl serum
	300 μl total volume

Read absorbance at one minute intervals for 5–10 minutes. If ΔA/min. is greater than 0.030/min., dilute serum with phosphate buffer and repeat measurements.

Calculations

ΔA/min. is obtained graphically (see page 41) or by calculating the mean.

Measurement at 366 nm

$$\frac{\Delta A}{3.3 \times 10^3} \times 10^6 \times \frac{300}{10} = \Delta A \times 9090 = \text{m}\mu\text{moles/min.} \times \text{ml}$$
$$= \text{mU/ml serum}$$

Measurement at 340 nm

$$\Delta A \times 4838 = \text{m}\mu\text{moles/min.} \times \text{ml} = \text{mU/ml serum}$$

Measurement at 334 nm

$$\Delta A \times 5000 = \text{m}\mu\text{moles/min.} \times \text{ml} = \text{mU/ml serum.}$$

For calculations with tan α see page 44.

If serum was diluted, the dilution factor has to be considered. With pipet volumes different from those prescribed, the factors must be recalculated (general formula on page 44).

Normal serum values: 48–96 mU/ml.

ALDOLASE (ALD)

Literature: Bruns, F., Biochem. z. **325**, 156 (1954); Beisenherz, G., H. J. Boltze, T. Bücher, R. Czok, K. H. Garbade, E. Meyer-Arendt, and G. Pfleiderer, Z. Naturforsch. **8b**, 555 (1953).

Principle

Aldolase catalyzes the reaction

$$\text{fructose-1,6-diphosphate} \rightleftharpoons \text{glyceraldehyde phosphate} + \text{dihydroxyacetone phosphate}$$

In the presence of triosephosphate isomerase (TIM) the following equilibrium is 96% on the side of dihydroxyacetone-phosphate

$$\underset{4\%}{\text{glyceraldehyde phosphate}} \xrightleftharpoons{\text{TIM}} \underset{96\%}{\text{dihydroxyacetone phosphate}}$$

Glycerophosphate dehydrogenase (GDH) with NADH reduces dihydroxyacetone phosphate to glycerol-3-phosphate

$$2 \text{ dihydroxyacetone phosphate} + 2 \text{ NADH} + H^+ \xrightleftharpoons{\text{GDH}} 2 \text{ glycerol-3-phosphate} + 2 \text{ NAD}^+$$

Overall reaction:

$$\text{fructose-1,6-diphosphate} + 2 \text{ NADH} + H^+ \rightleftharpoons 2 \text{ glycerol-3-phosphate} + 2 \text{ NAD}^+$$

NADH is oxidized in equimolar amounts and the rate of oxidation is the parameter of the aldolase activity.

Reagents

A. *Collidine buffer* 0.05M, pH 7.4 with *fructose-1,6-diphosphate* 2×10^{-3}M and *monoiodoacetate* 3×10^{-4}M: dissolve 8.56 mg fructose-1,6-diphosphate (Na-salt) and 0.63 mg monoiodoacetate (Na-salt) in 10.0 ml collidine buffer.

B. *NADH solution* 1.5×10^{-2}M: dissolve 10.6 mg NADH-Na_2 in 1.0 ml collidine buffer pH 7.4. Note the purity of the NADH sample and increase the amount of substance if necessary.

C. *GDH/TIM solution:* approximate activity required GDH 70 U/ml. TIM 500 U/ml. Suspend 2 mg GDH/TIM (mixed crystals) in 1 ml ammoniun sulfate solution 2.8M. Crystalline suspensions are commercially available from Sigma, St. Louis, Missouri, and Boehringer-Mannheim Corp., New York, New York.

Procedure

Required amount of serum: 20 μl, fresh and free from visible hemolysis.
Wavelength: 366, 340 or 334 nm; incubation temperature: 37°C.
Pipet into a 10-mm microcuvette

	274 μl buffered substrate (A)
	5 μl NADH (B)
	1 μl GDH/TIM (C)
Mix with plastic stirrer and preincubate for 5 minutes at 37°C; then add	
	20 μl serum
	300 μl total volume

Mix with plastic stirrer and read absorbance at 5 minute intervals for at least 20 minutes. Because of the normally low activity of ALD in serum, incubation is carried out at 37°C. If a temperature-controlled cuvette holder is not available, the cuvettes are kept in a water bath between readings. In case of a high self-absorption of serum, a blank is prepared containing 280 μl 0.9% saline and 20 μl serum. If not enough serum is available, prepare a blank as suggested on page 42. The difference in absorbance between sample and blank should initially be at least 0.5 but not more than 0.8.

Calculation

ΔA/min. is obtained graphically (see page 41) or by calculating the mean.

Measurement at 366 nm:

$$\frac{\Delta A}{3.3 \times 10^3} \times 10^6 \times \frac{300}{20} \times 0.5 = \Delta A \times 2273 = \text{m}\mu\text{moles/min.} \times \text{ml} = \text{mU/ml serum}$$

Measurement at 340 nm:

$$\Delta A \times 1210 = \text{m}\mu\text{moles/min.} \times \text{ml} = \text{mU/ml serum.}$$

Measurement at 334 nm:

$$\Delta A \times 1250 = \text{m}\mu\text{moles/min.} \times \text{ml} = \text{mU/ml serum}$$

The temperature coefficient for aldolase is 12% per 1°C. If the measurements were made at 37 °C, the values have to be multiplied by 0.41 to obtain the activity at 25 °C. Hence:

at 366 nm $\Delta A \times 931.5 =$ mU/ml serum
at 340 nm $\Delta A \times 496 =$ mU/ml serum
at 334 nm $\Delta A \times 512.5 =$ mU/ml serum

For calculation with tan α see page 44.
With pipet volumes different from those prescribed, the factors must be recalculated (general formula on page 44).

Normal serum values: 1.0–2.5 mU/ml.

GLUTAMATE OXALACETATE TRANSAMINASE (GOT)

Literature: Karmen, A., F. W. Wroblewski, and I. S. LaDue: J. Clin. Invest. **34**, 126 (1955).

Principle

GOT catalyzes the reaction.

$$\text{glutamate} + \text{oxaloacetate} \rightleftharpoons \text{aspartate} + \text{2-oxoglutarate}$$

In the reaction, proceeding from right to left, the rate of formation of oxaloacetate is measured with an indicator reaction catalyzed by malate dehydrogenase (MDH).

$$\text{oxaloacetate} + \text{NADH} + \text{H}^+ \xrightleftharpoons{\text{MDH}} \text{malate} + \text{NAD}^+$$

NADH is oxidized in equimolar amounts and the rate of oxidation is a measure for the activity of GOT.

Reagents

A. *Phosphate buffer* 0.1M, pH 7.4 with *Na-L-aspartate* 4.2×10^{-2}M: dissolve 72.7 mg Na-aspartate in 10 ml buffer.

B. *2-Oxoglutarate solution* 0.2M: dissolve 29.2 mg 2-oxoglutaric acid in 1 ml 0.40N NaOH.

C. *NADH solution* 1.2×10^{-2}M: dissolve 8.5 mg NADH-Na_2 in 1.0 ml phosphate buffer. Note the purity of the NADH sample and increase the amount of substance if necessary.

D. *Malate dehydrogenase* (MDH): minimum activity 700 U/mg. In 0.5 ml redistilled water dissolve 0.5 mg MDH and add 0.5 ml glycerol. If a commercial suspension of MDH in ammonium sulfate solution is used, dialyze for 4 hours at 0°C against phosphate buffer, pH 7.6, and dilute with glycerol to give 50% (w/v) glycerol and 0.5 mg enzyme protein/ml.

Procedure

Required amount of serum: 50 µl, fresh and free from visible hemolysis. Wavelength: 366, 340 or 334 nm; incubation temperature: 25°C.

Pipet into a 10-mm microcuvette

230 µl buffered aspartate (A)
5 µl NADH (C)
5 µl MDH (D)
50 µl serum

Mix with polyethylene stirrer and incubate for 15 minutes at 25°C in a water bath or directly in a tempertature-controlled cuvette holder. Endogenous metabolites in serum (pyruvate, oxaloacetate, etc.) will react with enzymes in serum with consumption of NADH. When no further change in absorbance occurs, add

10 μl 2-oxoglutarate (B)

300 μl total volume

Mix with polyethylene stirrer and read absorbance at one minute intervals for 5–10 minutes. In case of a high self-absorption of the serum (>0.800), a blank is prepared containing 250 μl 0.9% saline and 50 μl serum. If not enough serum is available, prepare a blank as suggested on page 42. ΔA/min. should not exceed 0.040. Dilute highly active sera with buffered aspartate (A). MDH preparations may contain traces of GOT. This activity is determined once for each sample by substituting redistilled water (with 0.2 μg pyridoxal phosphate/ml) for serum. Any "blank" activity is subtracted from the activity in serum.

Calculation

ΔA/min. is obtained graphically (see page 44) or by calculating the mean.

Measurement at 366 nm:

$$\frac{\Delta A}{3.3 \times 10^3} \times 10^6 \times \frac{300}{50} = \Delta A \times 1818 = \text{m}\mu\text{moles/min.} \times \text{ml} = \text{mU/ml serum}$$

Measurement at 340 nm:

$$\Delta A \times 968 = \text{m}\mu\text{moles/min.} \times \text{ml} = \text{mU/ml serum}$$

Measurement at 334 nm:

$$\Delta A \times 1000 = \text{m}\mu\text{moles/min.} \times \text{ml} = \text{mU/ml serum}$$

For calculation with tan α see page 44.
If the serum was diluted, the dilution factor has to be considered.
With pipet volumes different from those prescribed, the factors must be recalculated (general formula on page 44).

Normal serum values: 5–12 mU/ml.

GLUTAMATE PYRUVATE TRANSAMINASE (GPT)

Literature: Wroblewski, F., Clin. Chem. **2**, 250 (1956).

Principle

GPT catalyzes the reaction

$$\text{glutamate} + \text{pyruvate} \rightleftharpoons \text{alanine} + \text{2-oxoglutarate}$$

In the reaction proceeding from right to left, the rate of formation of pyruvate is measured with an indicator reaction catalyzed by lactate dehydrogenase (LDH).

$$\text{pyruvate} + \text{NADH} + \text{H}^+ \xrightleftharpoons{\text{(LDH)}} \text{lactate} + \text{NAD}^+$$

NADH is oxidized in equimolar amounts and the rate of oxidation is a measure for the activity of GPT.

Reagents

A. *Phosphate buffer* 0.1M, pH 7.4, with *alanine* 8.5×10^{-2}M: dissolve 0.94 g D,L-alanine (Na-salt) in 100 ml buffer.
B. *2-Oxoglutarate solution* 0.2M: dissolve 29.2 mg 2-oxoglutaric acid in 1 ml 0.4N NaOH.
C. *NADH solution*, 1.2×10^{-2}M: dissolve 8.5 mg NADH-Na_2 in 1.0 ml phosphate buffer. Note the purity of the NADH sample and increase the amount of substance if necessary.
D. *Lactate dehydrogenase* (LDH): minimum activity 300 U/mg. Dissolve 0.5 mg LDH in 0.5 ml redistilled water and add 0.5 ml glycerol. If a commercial suspension of LDH in ammonium sulfate solution is used, dialyze for 4 hours at 0°C against phosphate buffer, pH 7.6, and dilute with glycerol to give 50% (v/v) glycerol and 0.5 mg enzyme protein/ml.

Procedure

Required amount of serum: 50 μl, fresh and free from visible hemolysis. Wavelength 366, 340 or 334 nm; incubation temperature: 25°C.

Pipet into a 10-mm microcuvette

230 μl buffered alanine (A)
5 μl NADH (B)
5 μl LDH (D)
50 μl serum

Mix with polyethylene stirrer and incubate for 15 minutes at 25°C in water bath or directly in temperature-controlled cuvette holder. Endogenous metabolites in serum (pyruvate, oxaloacetate, etc.) will react with enzymes in serum with consumption of NADH. When no further change in absorbance occurs, add

10 μl 2-oxoglutarate (B)

300 μl total volume

Mix with polyethylene stirrer and read absorbance at one minute intervals for 5–10 minutes. In case of a high self-absorption of serum (>0.800), a blank is prepared containing 250 μl 0.9% saline and 50 μl serum. If not enough serum is available, prepare blank as suggested on page 42. ΔA/min. should not exceed 0.040. Dilute highly active sera with buffered alanine (A).

Calculation

ΔA/min. is obtained graphically (see page 41) or by calculating the mean.

Measurement at 366 nm:

$$\frac{\Delta A}{3.3 \times 10^3} \times 10^6 \times \frac{300}{50} = \Delta A \times 1818 = \text{m}\mu\text{moles/min.} \times \text{ml}$$
$$= \text{mU/ml serum}$$

Measurement at 340 nm:

$$\Delta A \times 968 = \text{m}\mu\text{moles/min.} \times \text{ml} = \text{mU/ml serum}$$

Measurement at 334 nm:

$$\Delta A \times 1000 = \text{m}\mu\text{moles/min.} \times \text{ml} = \text{mU/ml serum.}$$

For calculation with tan α see page 44.

If serum was diluted, the dilution factor has to be considered. With pipet volumes different from those prescribed, the factors must be recalculated (general formula on page 44).

Normal serum values: 5–12 mU/ml

GLUTAMATE DEHYDROGENASE (GLDH)

Literature: Pfleiderer, G., in H. M. Rauen, Biochemisches Taschenbuch (Berlin-Göttingen-Heidelberg: Springer-Verlag, 1956), p. 991; Schmidt, E., in H. U. Bergmeyer, Methods of Enzymatic Analysis (New York: Academic Press, 1963), p. 752.

Principle

GLDH catalyzes the reaction

$$\text{glutamate} + H_2O + NAD^+ \rightleftharpoons \text{2-oxoglutarate} + NH_4^+ + NADH + H^+$$

Under the experimental conditions the equilibrium is on the side of glutamate and NAD^+. NADH is oxidized in equimolar amounts and the rate of oxidation is a measure of the enzyme activity.

Reagents

A. *Triethanolamine buffer* 0.05M, pH 8.0, with 0.004M *EDTA*: dissolve 77 mg disodium dihydrogen ethylenediaminetetraacetate-$Na_2H_2 \times 2\ H_2O$ in 50.0 ml of buffer.
B. *Ammonium acetate solution*, 1.5M: dissolve 1.17 g ammonium acetate in 10 ml redistilled water.
C. *2-Oxoglutarate solution* 0.1M: dissolve 14.6 mg 2-oxoglutaric acid in 1 ml 0.2N NaOH.
D. *NADH solution* 5×10^{-3}M: dissolve 3.55 mg NADH-Na_2 in 1 ml triethanolamine buffer. Note purity of NADH sample and increase amount if necessary.

Procedure

Required amount of serum: 50 μl. Wavelength: 366, 340 or 334 nm; incubation temperature: 25°C.

Pipet into a 10-mm microcuvette

	200 μl buffer (A) 10 μl NADH (D) 20 μl NH_4AC (B) 50 μl serum
Mix with polyethylene stirrer and incubate for 10 minutes at 25°C in water bath or directly in temperature-controlled cuvette	

holder. Endogenous substrates (pyruvate, oxaloacetate, etc.) will react with enzymes in serum with consumption of NADH. When no further change in absorbance occurs, add

20 μl 2-oxoglutarate (C)

300 μl total volume

Mix with polyethylene stirrer and read absorbance at one minute intervals for 5–10 minutes. In case of high self-absorption of serum (>0.800), a blank is prepared containing 250 μl 0.9% saline and 50 μl serum. If not enough serum is available, prepare blank as suggested on page 42.

Calculation

ΔA/min. is obtained graphically (see page 41) or by calculating the mean.

Measurement at 366 nm:

$$\frac{\Delta A}{3.3 \times 10^3} \times 10^6 \times \frac{300}{50} = \Delta A \times 1818 = \text{m}\mu\text{moles/min} = \text{mU/ml serum}$$

Measurement at 340 nm:

$$\Delta A \times 968 = \text{m}\mu\text{moles/min.} \times \text{ml} = \text{mU/ml serum}$$

Measurement at 334 nm:

$$\Delta A \times 1000 = \text{m}\mu\text{moles/min.} \times \text{ml} = \text{mU/ml serum.}$$

For calculation with tan α see page 44.
With pipet volumes different from those prescribed, the factors must be recalculated (general formula on page 44).

Normal serum values: below 0.9 mU/ml.

ISOCITRATE DEHYDROGENASE (ICDH)

Literature: Wolfson, S. K., and H. G. Williams-Ashman, Proc. Soc. Exp. Biol. Med. 96, 231 (1957); C. F. Boehringer, Mannheim: Technical Bulletin 1966.

Principle

ICDH catalyzes the reaction

$$\text{Isocitrate} + \text{NADP}^+ \xrightleftharpoons{\text{Mn}^{++}} \text{2-oxoglutarate} + \text{NADPH} + \text{H}^+ + \text{CO}_2$$

Under the experimental conditions the equilibrium is on the right side. NADP is reduced in equimolar amounts and the rate of reduction is a measure of the enzyme activity.

Reagents

A. *Triethanolamine buffer* 0.1M, pH 7.5, with D,L-*isocitrate* 4.6×10^{-3}M and *NaCl* 5.2×10^{-2}M: dissolve in 10 ml buffer 11.9 mg D,L-isocitrate (Na_3-salt) and 30.4 mg NaCl.

B. *$MnSO_4$ solution* 0.24M: dissolve 40.6 mg $MnSO_4 \times H_2O$ in 1 ml redistilled water.

C. *NADP solution* 1.82×10^{-2}M: dissolve 13.9 mg NADP-NaH_2 in 1 ml redistilled water.

Procedure

Required amount of serum: 50 μl, free from visible hemolysis.
Wavelength: 366, 340 or 334 nm; incubation temperature 25°C.
Pipet into a 10-mm microcuvette

	250 μl buffered isocitrate (A)
	50 μl serum
Mix with polyethylene stirrer and allow to stand for about 5 minutes. Then add	
	5 μl $MnSO_4$ (B)
	5 μl NADP (C)
	310 μl total volume

Mix and read absorbance at one minute intervals for about 10 minutes.

Calculation

ΔA/min. is obtained graphically (see page 41) or by calculating the mean.

Measurement at 366 nm:

$$\frac{\Delta A}{3.3 \times 10^3} \times 10^6 \times \frac{310}{50} = \Delta A \times 1878 = \text{m}\mu\text{moles/min.} \times \text{ml}$$
$$= \text{mU/ml serum}$$

Measurement at 340 nm:

$$\Delta A \times 1000 = \text{m}\mu\text{moles/min.} \times \text{ml} = \text{mU/ml serum}$$

Measurement at 334 nm:

$$\Delta A \times 1034 = \text{m}\mu\text{moles/min.} \times \text{ml} = \text{mU/ml serum}$$

For calculation with tan α see page 44. With pipet volumes different from those prescribed, the factors must be recalculated (general formula on page 44).

Normal serum values:

adults 0.6–5 mU/ml
newborn infants 3–8 mU/ml.

LACTATE DEHYDROGENASE (LDH)

Literature: Beisenherz, G., H. J. Boltze, T. Bücher, R. Czok, K. H. Garbade, E. Meyer-Arendt, and G. Pfleiderer, Z. Naturforsch. **8b**, 555 (1953); Bergmeyer, H. U., E. Bernt, and B. Hess, in H. U. Bergmeyer, Methods of Enzymatic Analysis (New York: Academic Press, 1963), p. 736.

Principle

Lactate dehydrogenase catalyzes the reaction

$$\text{lactate} + NAD^+ \rightleftharpoons \text{pyruvate} + NADH + H^+$$

Under the experimental conditions the equilibrium is far to the side of NAD and lactate. NADH is oxidized in equimolar amounts and the rate of oxidation is a measure of the enzyme activity.

Reagents

A. *Phosphate buffer* 0.05M, pH 7.5 with *pyruvate* 3×10^{-4}M: dissolve 3.3 mg Na-pyruvate in 100 ml buffer.

B. *NADH solution* 9.0×10^{-3}M: dissolve 6.38 mg NADH-Na_2 in 1.0 ml phosphate buffer, pH 7.5. Observe the purity indicated on the package and increase the amount of substance if necessary.

Procedure

Required amount of serum: 10 μl, fresh and free from visible hemolysis.
Wavelength: 366, 340 or 334 nm; incubation temperature: 25°C.
Pipet into a 10-mm microcuvette

300 μl	buffered pyruvate (A)
5 μl	NADH (B)
10 μl	serum
315 μl	total volume

Mix with polyethylene stirrer and read absorbance at one minute intervals for 3–5 minutes. ΔA/min. should not exceed 0.020/min. Dilute highly active sera 1:10 with buffered pyruvate (A).

Calculation

ΔA/min. is obtained graphically (see page 41) or by calculating the mean.

Measurement at 366 nm:

$$\frac{\Delta A}{3.3 \times 10^3} \times 10^6 \times \frac{315}{10} = \Delta A \times 9545 = \text{m}\mu\text{moles/min.} \times \text{ml}$$
$$= \text{mU/ml serum}$$

Measurement at 340 nm:

$$\Delta A \times 5080 = \text{m}\mu\text{moles/min.} \times \text{ml} = \text{mU/ml serum}$$

Measurement at 334 nm:

$$\Delta A \times 5250 = \text{m}\mu\text{moles/min.} \times \text{ml} = \text{mU/ml serum}$$

For calculation with tan α see page 44. If serum was diluted, the dilution factor has to be considered. With pipet volumes different from those prescribed, the factors must be recalculated (general formula on page 44).

Normal serum values: up to 180 mU/ml

1-PHOSPHOFRUCTALDOLASE (PFA)

Literature: Wolf, H. P., G. Forster, and F. Leuthardt, Gastroenterologia **87**, 172 (1957).

Principle

1-Phosphofructaldolase catalyzes the reaction

$$\text{fructose-1-phosphate} \rightleftharpoons \text{glyceraldehyde} + \text{dihydroxyacetone phosphate}$$

In the presence of glycerolphosphate dehydrogenase (GDH) and NADH, dihydroxyacetone phosphate reacts further

$$\text{dihydroxyacetone phosphate} + \text{NADH} + \text{H}^+ \xrightleftharpoons{\text{GDH}} \text{glycerol-3-phosphate} + \text{NAD}^+$$

NADH is oxidized in amounts proportional to the consumption of fructose-1-phosphate and the rate of oxidation is a measure of the activity of 1-phosphofructaldolase.

Reagents

A. *NADH solution* 1.5×10^{-2}M: dissolve 10.6 mg NADH-Na_2 in 1 ml 1% $NaHCO_3$ solution. Note purity of the NADH sample and increase amount if necessary.

B. *Fructose-1-phosphate solution* 0.2M: dissolve 917 mg fructose-1-phosphate dicyclohexylammonium salt in 10 ml redistilled water.

C. *Glycerolphosphate dehydrogenase*: minimum activity 30 U/mg. Use commercially available crystalline suspension in ammonium sulfate solution with 2 mg protein/ml.

Procedure

Required amount of serum: 180 μl.
No buffer is necessary because the buffering capacity of serum is sufficient. Wavelength: 366, 340 or 334 nm; incubation temperature: 25°C.

Pipet into a 10-mm microcuvette

180 μl serum
5 μl NADH (A)

Mix with polyethlene stirrer and incubate for 20 minutes at 25°C in water bath or directly in temperature-controlled cuvette holder. Endogenous metabolites in serum (pyruvate, oxaloacetate, etc.) react with enzymes in serum with consumption of NADH. When no further change in absorbance occurs, add

1 μl GDH (C)
20 μl fructose-1-phosphate (B)
206 μl total volume

Mix with polyethylene stirrer. Wait for about 5 minutes before reading the absorbance because in the beginning the reaction is often not linear. Then read at 2–3 minute intervals until the total change in absorbance is at least 0.050. Read against a blank with 180 μl serum and 20 μl H_2O. If not enough serum is available, prepare blank as suggested on page 42.

Calculation

ΔA/min. is obtained graphically (see page 41) or by calculation of the mean.

Measurement at 366 nm:

$$\frac{\Delta A}{3.3 \times 10^3} \times 10^6 \times \frac{206}{180} = \Delta A \times 347 = \text{m}\mu\text{moles/min.} \times \text{ml} = \text{mU/ml serum}$$

Measurement at 340 nm:

$$\Delta A \times 184 = \text{m}\mu\text{moles/min.} \times \text{ml} = \text{mU/ml serum}$$

Measurement at 334 nm:

$$\Delta A \times 191 = \text{m}\mu\text{moles/min.} \times \text{ml} = \text{mU/ml serum}$$

For calculation with tan α see page 44. With pipet volumes different from those prescribed, the factors must be recalculated (general formula on page 44).

Normal serum values: < 1 mU/ml

PHOSPHOHEXOSE ISOMERASE (PHI)

Literature: Bruns, F., and K. Hinsberg, Biochem. Z. **325**, 532 (1954).

Principle

Phosphohexose isomerase catalyzes the reversible reaction

$$\text{glucose-6-phosphate} \rightleftharpoons \text{fructose-6-phosphate}$$

The amount of fructose-6-phosphate formed per unit time is measured. Fructose-6-phosphate reacts with resorcinol in hydrochloric acid to form a reddish color complex which is determined colorimetrically.

Reagents

A. *Veronal buffer* 0.1M, pH 7.8.

B. *Glucose-6-phosphate solution* 0.06M, pH 7.8: dissolve 182 mg glucose-6-phosphate (Na-salt) in 10 ml Veronal buffer (A).

C. *Trichloroacetic acid* (TCA) 7%

D. *Resorcinol solution*: 1% in ethanol

E. *HCl,* 30%

Procedure

Required amount of serum: 2 × 20 μl
Pipet into a micro test tube

	20 μl serum
	20 μl buffer (A)
	20 μl glucose-6-ph (B)
Mix with vibrator and incubate for 30–60 minutes at 37°C, then add	
	140 μl TCA (C)
Mix and centrifuge. Pipet into a micro test tube	
	40 μl clear supernatant
	40 μl resorcinol (D)
	120 μl HCl (E)

Mix and incubate for 8 minutes at 80°C, cool for 5 minutes in water bath at room temperature. Read absorbance in 10-mm microcuvette at 490 nm against a serum blank to which glucose-6-phosphate (B) was added after TCA, but which was treated identically otherwise.

Calculation

The activity is calculated from a calibration curve constructed with fructose-6-phosphate. Bruns and Hinsberg express the activity in mm^3 fructose-6-phosphate formed per ml serum per hour (1 μmole fructose-6-phosphate = 260 μg = 22.4 mm^3).

Normal values: 86–112 mm^3 fructose-6-phosphate/ml serum = 64–83 mU/ml serum.

SORBITOL DEHYDROGENASE (SDH)

Literature: Holzer, H., J. Haan, and S. Schneider, Biochem. Z. **326**, 451 (1955); Gerlach, U., and E. Schürmeyer, Z. Ges. Exp. Med. **132**, 413 (1960).

Principle

Sorbitol dehydrogenase catalyzes the reaction

$$\text{sorbitol} + \text{NAD}^+ \rightleftharpoons \text{fructose} + \text{NADH} + \text{H}^+$$

Under the experimental conditions the equilibrium is to the side of sorbitol and NAD^+. NADH is oxidized in equimolar quantities and the rate of oxidation is a measure of the enzyme activity.

Reagents

A. *Triethanolamine buffer* 0.2M, pH 7.4
B. *Fructose solution* 72% (w/v)
C. *NADH solution* 1.0×10^{-2}M: dissolve 7.1 mg NADH-Na_2 in 1 ml buffer (A). Note the purity of the NADH sample and increase the amount if necessary.

Procedure

Required amount of serum: 50 μl
Wavelength: 366, 340 or 334 nm; incubation temperature: 25°C.
Pipet into a 10-mm microcuvette

	125 μl buffer (A)
	50 μl serum
	5 μl NADH (C)
Mix with polyethylene stirrer and incubate for 10 minutes at 25°C in water bath or directly in temperature-controlled cuvette holder. Endogenous metabolites (pyruvate, oxaloacetate, etc.) react with enzymes in serum with consumption of NADH. When no further change in absorbance occurs, add	
	20 μl fructose (B)
	200 μl total volume

Mix with polyethylene stirrer and read absorbance at one minute intervals for about 10 minutes. In case of high self-absorption of serum (>.800), a blank is prepared containing 150 μl saline and 50 μl serum. If not enough serum is available, prepare blank as suggested on page 42.

Calculation

ΔA/min. is obtained graphically (see page 41) or by calculating the mean.

Measurement at 366 nm:

$$\frac{\Delta A}{3.3 \times 10^3} \times 10^6 \times \frac{200}{50} = \Delta A \times 1212 = \text{m}\mu\text{moles/min.} \times \text{ml}$$
$$= \text{mU/ml serum}$$

Measurement at 340 nm:

$\Delta A \times 645 = \text{m}\mu\text{moles/min.} \times \text{ml} = \text{mU/ml serum}$

Measurement at 334 nm:

$\Delta A \times 667 = \text{m}\mu\text{moles/min.} \times \text{ml} = \text{mU/ml serum}$

For calculation with tan α see page 44. With pipet volumes different from those prescribed, the factors must be recalculated (general formula on page 44).

Normal serum values: < 1 mU/ml

α-AMYLASE

Literature: Street, H. V., and J. R. Close, Clin. Chim. Acta **1**, 256 (1956) (micromethod).

Principle

α-Amylase degrades amylose to dextrins and a mixture of reducing saccharides. The difference in color intensity after addition of iodine to amylose before and after enzymatic hydrolysis is measured.

Reagents

A. *Amylose solution* 0.1%: suspend 100 mg amylose in 5 ml ethanol and pour into about 70 ml 0.01N NaOH heated to about 90°C. Rinse traces of amylose from the container into the hot NaOH with two 1-ml portions of ethanol. Most of the ethanol boils off. Cool solution, transfer to a volumetric flask and add 0.01N NaOH to 100 ml. Mix well and store at room temperature.
B. *Phosphate buffer* 0.02M, pH 7.0
C. *NaCl solution* 0.85% (w/v)
D. *HCl* 0.01N
E. *Buffer-substrate mixture:* mix 2.5 ml phosphate buffer (B), 1 ml 0.01N HCl (D), 1.0 ml amylose solution (A), and 0.5 ml NaCl solution (C).
F. *Iodine-potassium iodide solution:* dissolve 3 g KI in 25 ml redistilled water, add 1.27 g iodine and bring to 100 ml. Store in the dark. Prior to use, dilute 1:10 with redistilled water.

Procedure

Required amount of serum: 5 μl Pipet into a 10-ml test tube with ground glass stopper	
	50 μl NaCl (C) 5 μl serum 500 μl buffer substrate (E)
Mix thoroughly and incubate for exactly 15 minutes at 37°C; then add	
	5 ml redistilled water 300 μl iodine solution (F)

Mix thoroughly and measure absorbance at 620 nm or nearby wavelength against water. The standard is prepared as above, replacing serum with redistilled water. If, after the addition of iodine solution, the color is not blue-green but violet, reddish or yellow, the amylase activity is too high. Repeat with serum diluted 1:5 or 1:10 with saline (C).

Calculation

A_S = absorbance of amylose standard
A_T = absorbance of sample

$$\frac{A_S - A_T}{A_S} \times 100 = \text{Street-Close units/100 ml serum.}$$

Multiply with dilution factor if serum was diluted.

$$(\text{Street-Close units/100 ml}) \times 5.7 = \text{mU/ml}$$

Normal value in serum (37°C): 6–33 Street-Close units/100 ml
34–188 mU/ml.

Remark

Fresh serum should be used because the activity of α-amylase decreases relatively quickly at room temperature. Serum may be kept at 4°C for 2–3 hours without significant loss of activity.

LEUCINE AMINOPEPTIDASE (LAP) (Arylaminopeptidase)

Method 1: Leucyl-β-naphthylamide as substrate.

Literature: Goldbarg, J. A., and A. M. Rutenburg, Cancer **11**, 283 (1958); Wust, H., in Methods of Enzymatic Analysis, H. U. Bergmeyer, editor (New York: Academic Press, second revised printing 1965), p. 830.

Principle

Leucine aminopeptidase catalyzes the reaction

L-Leucyl-β-naphthylamide + $H_2O \rightleftharpoons$ L-leucine + β-naphthylamine

The amount of β-naphthylamine liberated per unit time is proportional to the enzyme activity. β-Naphthylamine is diazotized and coupled with naphthylethylenediamine. The violet azo dye is measured colorimetrically.

Reagents

A. *Phosphate buffer* 0.1M, pH 7.2

B. L-*Leucyl-β-naphthylamide hydrochloride solution:* 0.2% (w/v) in methanol

C. *Perchloric acid ca.* 20% (w/v): dilute 17.5 ml 70% $HClO_4$ to 100 ml with redistilled water.

D. *Sodium nitrite solution* 0.2% (w/v): dissolve 20 mg $NaNO_2$ in 10 ml redistilled water.

E. *Ammonium sulfamate solution* 0.5% (w/v): dissolve 50 mg ammonium sulfamate in 10 ml redistilled water.

F. N-*(1-naphthyl)-ethylenediamine dihydrochloride solution* 0.05% (w/v): dissolve 5 mg of the dihydrochloride in 10 ml methanol.

G. *NaCl solution* 0.9%

β-naphthylamine standards:

(1) 50 mμg β-naphthylamine per μl: dissolve 6.275 mg β-naphthylamine hydrochloride in phosphate buffer (A) and bring to 100 ml.

(2) 5 mμg β-naphthylamine per μl: immediately before use dilute solution (1) 1:10 with phosphate buffer (A).

Procedure

Required amount of serum: 10 μl
Pipet into a micro test tube

	130 μl buffer (A) 40 μl saline (G) 10 μl serum 20 μl substrate (B)
Mix with vibrator and incubate for exactly 30 minutes at 37°C. Then add	
	100 μl perchloric acid (C)
Mix and centrifuge. Pipet into a micro test tube	
	100 μl supernatant 100 μl nitrite solution (D)
Mix and incubate for 10 minutes at 37°C. Then add	
	100 μl sulfamate solution (E)
Mix, and after 2 minutes add	
	200 μl naphthylethylenediamine solution (F)

Mix and incubate for 30 minutes at 37°C. Cool to room temperature and read absorbance at 580 nm or nearby wavelength in 10-mm microcuvettes against a reagent blank. The blank is treated like the sample but contains saline (G) instead of serum.

Calibration curve

Prepare six micro test tubes as follows:

	β-naphthylamine (mμg)	standard (1) μl	standard (2) μl	saline (G) μl	buffer (A) μl
1	100	—	20	50	130
2	250	—	50	50	100
3	500	—	100	50	50
4	1000	20	—	50	130
5	2500	50	—	50	100
6	0	—	—	50	150

Add 100 μl perchloric acid and proceed as described in above procedure. Read absorbance against #6. Plot absorbance over mμg β-naphthylamine.

Calculation

Read from standard curve the amount of β-napthylamine liberated by the sample

$$\text{m}\mu\text{g naphthylamine} \times \frac{100}{143.18 \times 30} = \text{m}\mu\text{moles/min.} \times \text{ml serum}$$
$$= \text{mU/ml serum}$$

mμg naphthylamine × 0.0233 = mU/ml serum

Where 100 = conversion to 1.0 ml serum (10 μl in test)
30 = incubation time in min.
143.18 = molecular weight of β-naphthylamine

Normal values: 18–37 mU/ml serum

Method 2: Leucine-p-nitroanilide as substrate

Literature: Tuppy, H., U. Wiesbauer, and E. Wintersberger, Z. Physiol. Chem. **329**, 278 (1962); Willig, F., I. Greinez, H. Stork, and F. H. Schmidt, Klin. Wochschr. **45**, 474 (1967).

Principle

Leucine aminopeptidase catalyzes the reaction

$$\text{L-Leucine-}p\text{-nitroanilide} + H_2O \rightleftharpoons \text{L-leucine} + p\text{-nitroaniline}$$

p-Nitroaniline can directly be measured photometrically at 380-410 nm.

Reagents

A. *Phosphate buffer* 0.05M, pH 7.2
B. *Leucine-p-nitroanilide solution* 0.025M: dissolve 19.2 mg L-leucine-*p*-nitroanilide in 3.0 ml methanol.
C. *Acetic acid* 30%

Procedure

Required amount of serum: 10 μl, fresh and free of visible hemolysis.

Pipet into a 10-mm microcuvette	300 μl buffer (A)
	10 μl substrate (B)
Mix with polyethylene stirrer and preincubate for 5 minutes at 25°C in water bath or directly in	

temperature-controlled cuvette
holder; then add

10 μl serum

320 μl total volume

Read absorbance (= A_1) at 405 nm, allow to stand at 25°C and read absorbance (= A_2) exactly 30 minutes after the first measurement. $\Delta A = A_2 - A_1$. With $\Delta A > 0.600$, dilute serum 1:10 with saline and repeat test. If a larger series has to be measured, incubate in micro test tubes. Exactly 30 minutes after serum has been added, stop reaction with 200 μl acetic acid (C). A separate blank, to which serum is added after acetic acid, must then be prepared for each serum. Read against these blanks.

LAP can also be measured in a kinetic test. Prepare microcuvette as above and read absorbance at 2–3 minute intervals. With $\Delta A/\text{min.} > 0.030$ dilute serum with saline and repeat test.

Calculation

p-Nitroaniline: $\varepsilon_{405} = 9.8765 \times 10^3$ (1/mole × cm)

(1) 30 minute incubation, no acetic acid

$$\Delta A = A_2 - A_1$$

$$\frac{\Delta A}{9.8765 \times 10^3} \times 10^6 \times \frac{1}{30} \times \frac{320}{10} = \Delta A \times 108 = \text{mU/ml}$$

(2) 30 minute incubation, with acetic acid

$$\frac{\Delta A}{9.8765 \times 10^3} \times 10^6 \times \frac{1}{30} \times \frac{520}{10} = \Delta A \times 175 = \text{mU/ml.}$$

(3) Kinetic test
Obtain ΔA/min. graphically or by calculation of the mean.

$$\frac{\Delta A/\text{min.}}{9.8765 \times 10^3} \times 10^6 \times \frac{320}{10} = \Delta A/\text{min.} \times 3240 = \text{mU/ml}$$

With pipet volumes different from those prescribed, the factors must be recalculated (general formula on page 44).
If measurement cannot be made at 405 nm, a standard curve must be prepared with *p*-nitroaniline.

Normal values: 8–22 mU/ml

LIPASE

Literature: Tietz, N. W., T. Borden, and J. D. Stepleton, Am. J. Clin. Pathol. **31**, 148 (1959).

Principle

Lipase hydrolyzes neutral fat to glycerol and fatty acids. The amount of fatty acids is determined by titration with NaOH. Accuracy and reproducibility depend on the stability of the fat emulsion. To avoid difficulties in this regard, water-soluble synthetic substrates have been introduced. These substrates, however, are hydrolyzed not only by lipase but by unspecific esterases as well. To measure the "true" lipase, Tietz *et al.* developed a method with a stable olive oil emulsion as substrate.

Reagents

A. *Stable olive oil emulsion*: to 93 ml redistilled water add 0.2 g Na-benzoate and 7 g Gum Arabic and homogenize in a Waring blendor at low speed. Still at low speed slowly add 93 ml olive oil (highest purity) and continue homogenization for another 3 minutes. Finally homogenize at high speed for 5 minutes. Store emulsion at 10–14°C for not longer than six months. Shake before use.

B. *Tris buffer* 0.2M, pH 8.0

C. *Indicator solution*: dissolve 100 mg thymolphthalein in 10 ml ethanol.

D. *Ethanol* 95%

E. *NaOH* 0.050N, carefully standardized. Store in polyethylene bottle.

Procedure

Required amount of serum: 10 μl for enzyme test and 10 μl for blank.

Pipet into a 30 × 4-mm micro test tube	25 μl H_2O 30 μl emulsion (A) 10 μl buffer (B) 10 μl serum
Close test tubes with Parafilm and mix intensively with vibrator for 10	

seconds. Incubate for 6 hours at
37°C; then add 30 μl ethanol (D)
1 μl indicator (C)

Mix and titrate with NaOH (see description of titration set in Figure 30). A blank containing water, emulsion and buffer must be run with each set of analyses. At the end of the incubation period add ethanol and indicator; mix in serum immediately prior to titration. Titrate blank to a distinct blue color first. Use blank for color comparison when titrating the samples.

Calculation

According to Tietz, Borden and Stepleton:

Lipase units = ml 0.050N NaOH required per 1.0 ml serum, or for microtest

Lipase units = μl 0.050N NaOH required per 1 μl of serum.

With 10 μl serum in test

$$\text{Lipase units} = \frac{\mu\text{l } 0.050\text{N NaOH}}{10}$$

Example:

NaOH required for sample	15.5 μl
NaOH required for blank	3.5 μl
	Δ = 12.0 μl

$$\frac{12.0}{10} = 1.2 \text{ lipase units}$$

Calculation in mU/ml (= mμmoles/ml × min.)

$$\frac{(\mu l_{\text{sample}} - \mu l_{\text{blank}}) \times [\text{NaOH}] \times 10^6}{\text{Incub. time (min.)} \times \text{serum volume } (\mu l)} = \text{mU/ml serum}$$

for the given example

$$\frac{12.0 \times 0.050 \times 10^6}{360 \times 10} = 167 \text{ mU/ml serum}$$

The factor 10^6 converts moles/L to mμmoles/ml.

Normal serum values:

0.5–1.5 lipase units
70–210 mU/ml

Titration set

- holder for 2 micro test tubes
- adjustable support
- electromagnet with contact breaker
- magnetic stirrers ("fleas" see page 24)
- microtitrator with polyethylene tubing attached to the tip of the titrator

The assembled set is shown in Figure 30.

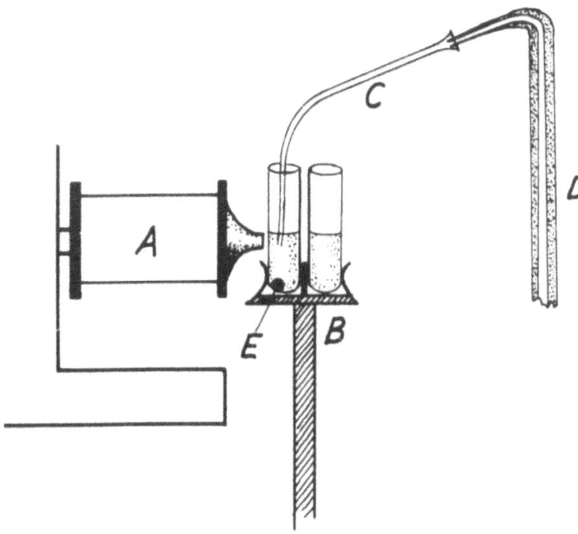

Figure 30. Microtitration assembly according to Linderstrøm-Lang and Holter.

(A) Electromagnet connected to an automatic circuit-breaker; (B) holder for micro test tubes, mounted on adjustable support; (C) polyethylene tube; (D) part of a microburet, *e.g.*, Beckman-Spinco 153-Microtitrator; (E) "flea."

Titration technique

Add one flea to each test tube. Insert test tubes with blank (next to magnet) and sample in holder. Adjust support to bring tip of magnet level with fluid surface in test tube. Start electromagnet; the flea will now move up and down. Lower tip of polyethylene tube into solution in blank test tube and immediately start to titrate slowly to a distinct blue color. Change test tubes and titrate sample to match the color of the blank. The test tube with the blank remains in the holder to serve for a color comparison in the titration of subsequent samples.

If an electromagnet is not available, the flea can be moved by hand with a small strong magnet. If a microtitrator is not available, add NaOH in 1 μl portions with a 1.0 μl constriction pipet. Naturally calculation in fractional units is not possible in this case.

ALKALINE PHOSPHATASE

Literature: Bessey, O. H., O. H., Lowry, and M. J. Brock, J. Biol. Chem. **164**, 321 (1946).

Principle

Alkaline phosphatase catalyzes the reaction

$$p\text{-nitrophenylphosphate} \longrightarrow \text{phosphate} + p\text{-nitrophenol}$$

The amount of *p*-nitrophenol liberated per unit time is directly proportional to the enzyme activity. *p*-Nitrophenol is measured photometrically in an alkaline solution.

Reagents

A. *Buffer*: dissolve 7.5. g glycine and 95 mg $MgCl_2$ in about 700 ml redistilled water, add 85 ml 1.0N NaOH and bring to 1000 ml, pH 10.3–10.4, check with glass electrode and correct if necessary.
B. *Substrate solution*: 0.4% solution of *p*-nitrophenylphosphate (disodium salt) in 0.001N HCl. Check for free *p*-nitrophenol in preparation: to 0.1 ml substrate solution add 1.0 ml 0.02N NaOH (D) and measure absorbance in 10-mm cuvette at 400 nm. If $A > 0.08$ recrystallize preparation from 87% ethanol.
C. *Buffer substrate mixture:* mix equal volumes of A and B.
D. *NaOH* 0.02N

Procedure

Required amount of serum: 5 μl for enzyme test, 5 μl for blank
Pipet into a micro test tube

5 μl serum
50 μl buffered substrate (C)

Mix with vibrator and incubate
for 30 minutes at 37°C; then add

500 μl NaOH (D)

Mix and read absorbance in 10-mm microcuvette at 400 nm against a blank to which serum was added after NaOH. If absorbance is above 0.800, dilute serum 1:10 with physiol. saline and multiply result by 10.

Calculation

The molar extinction coefficient of *p*-nitrophenol in alkaline solution at 400 nm is $\varepsilon = 18.8 \times 10^3$ (1/mole × cm).

$$\frac{A}{18.8 \times 10^3} \times 10^6 \times \frac{555}{5} \times \frac{1}{30} = A \times 197 = \text{m}\mu\text{moles/min.} \times \text{ml}$$
$$= \text{mU/ml serum}$$

at 405 nm: A × 201 = mU/ml serum.

For measurement at other wavelengths, construct a standard curve with *p*-nitrophenol. With pipet volumes different from those prescribed, the factor must be recalculated (general formula on page 44).

Normal values: 8–50 mU/ml serum (37°C).

Acid phosphatase

Proceed as described for alkaline phosphatase but replace the glycine buffer (A) with citrate buffer 0.05M, pH 4.8.

Normal values: 3–11 mU/ml serum

5-PHOSPHORIBOSE ISOMERASE

Literature: Bruns, H., Biochem. Z. **327**, 523 (1956).

Principle

5-Phosphoribose isomerase catalyzes the reversible reaction

$$\text{ribose-5-phosphate} \rightleftharpoons \text{ribulose-5-phosphate}$$

The rate of ribulose-5-phosphate formation is determined colorimetrically with Dische's carbazole reaction.

Reagents

A. *Tris buffer* 0.1M, pH 7.5
B. *Ribose-5-phosphate solution* 3×10^{-2}M: dissolve 72.2 mg ribose-5-phosphate (disodium salt) in 10 ml redistilled water.
C. *Trichloroacetic acid* (TCA) 10%
D. *H_2SO_4:* to 95 ml H_2O add 225 ml conc. H_2SO_4.
E. *Cysteine hydrochloride solution* 1.5%
F. *Carbazole solution* 0.12% in absolute ethanol.

Procedure

Required amount of serum: 10 μl (+ 10 μl for blank).
Pipet into a micro test tube

	10 μl serum 10 μl H_2O 20 μl buffer (A) 20 μl ribose-5-ph (B)
Mix with vibrator and incubate at 37°C for 10 minutes; then add	60 μl TCA (C)
Mix and centrifuge. Pipet into a micro test tube	
Do not change the sequence of addition.	50 μl clear supernatant 300 μl H_2SO_4 (D) 10 μl cysteine (E) 10 μl carbazole (F)

Complete addition of reagents within 40 seconds. Mix with vibrator. Incubate for 3 hours at 37°C, at which time the development of a red-violet color reaches the maximum. Cool to room temperature and read absorbance at 540 nm in a 10-mm microcuvette against a blank which was treated in the same way except that ribose-5-ph (B) was added *after* TCA (C).

Calculation

The calculation is based on a standard curve with ribulose-5-phosphate. Bruns defines 1 enzyme unit as the amount of ribulose-5-phosphate in μmoles (1 μmole = 230 μg) formed from ribose-5-phosphate by 1 ml serum per hour at pH 7.5 and 37°C. The construction of a standard curve is desirable but ribulose-5-phosphate is not yet commercially available. The factor given below was calculated from a standard curve published by Bruns, and can be used if the determination is carried out exactly as described.

$A_{540\ nm}^{10\ mm} = 0.100 = 1.8$ μmoles ribulose-5-phosphate/ml serum × hour

$A_{540\ nm}^{10\ mm} \times 18 =$ μmoles ribulose-5-phosphate/ml serum × hour

$A_{540\ nm}^{10\ mm} \times 18 \times 16.7 =$ mμmoles/ml × min. = mU/ml serum

Mean values for normal serum: 3.5 μmoles/ml × hour = 58.5 mU/ml

CREATINE PHOSPHOKINASE (CPK)

Literature: Tanzer, M. L. and C. Gilvarg, J. Biol. Chem. **234**, 3201 (1959).

Principle

CPK catalyzes the reversible reaction

$$\text{creatine} + \text{ATP} \rightleftharpoons \text{creatine phosphate} + \text{ADP}$$

The activity is measured with creatine and ATP by determining the rate of ADP formation. ADP is phosphorylated to ATP with phosphoenol pyruvate (PEP) and pyruvate kinase (PK) in the auxiliary reaction

$$\text{ADP} + \text{PEP} \xrightleftharpoons{\text{(PK)}} \text{ATP} + \text{pyruvate}$$

The pyruvate is determined with NADH and lactate dehydrogenase (LDH) in the indicator reaction

$$\text{pyruvate} + \text{NADH} + \text{H}^+ \xrightleftharpoons{\text{(LDH)}} \text{lactate} + \text{NAD}^+$$

NADH is oxidized in equimolar amounts and the rate of oxidation is a measure for the CPK activity.

Reagents

A. *Glycine buffer* 2.0M, pH 9.0 with *NADH* 1×10^{-3}M, *ATP* 6×10^{-3}M, *PEP* 2×10^{-3}M and *$MgSO_4$* 2×10^{-2}M: in 10 ml redistilled water dissolve 1.50 g glycine, 0.45 g Na_2CO_3, 7.1 mg NADH-Na_2 (note purity of sample and increase amount if necessary), 36.3 mg ATP-Na_2–$H_2 \times 3\ H_2O$, 9.3 mg PEP (cyclohexylammonium salt) and 26.7 mg $MgSO_4 \times 7\ H_2O$. When stored at 4°C the solution is stable for one week.

B. *Lactate dehydrogenase/pyruvate kinase* (LDH/PK): minimum activity: LDH 300 U/mg, PK 120 U/mg. Dilute commercial crystalline suspensions of LDH and PK with 2.2M ammonium sulfate to 4 mg protein/ml and mix equal parts of the suspensions.

C. *Buffer-substrate solution:* glycine buffer 0.1M, pH 9.0 with 6.3×10^{-2}M creatine. In 20 ml redistilled water, dissolve 150 mg glycine, 45 mg Na_2CO_3 and 175 mg creatine.

D. *Glycine buffer* 0.1M, pH 9.0: dissolve 150 mg glycine and 45 mg Na_2CO_3 in 20 ml redistilled water.

Procedure

Required amount of serum: 50 μl for enzyme test and 50 μl for serum blank.

Pipet into each of two 10 mm microcuvettes (enzyme test + blank)

	50 μl serum
	35 μl glycine buffer (A)
	3 μl LDH/PK (B)

Mix with polyethylene stirrer and incubate for 10 minutes at 25°C. Pyruvate and ADP, contained in PEP and ATP respectively, react with consumption of NADH. Then add

enzyme test:	90 μl buffer substrate (C)
blank:	90 μl buffer (D)
	178 μl total volume

With the blank in the light path, adjust abdorbance to 0.300 and then read enzyme test absorbance (= A_1). After exactly 10 minutes readjust blank to A = 0.300 and read enzyme test absorbance (= A_2). If a temperature-controlled cuvette holder is not available, cuvettes must be placed in a 25°C water bath during the 10 minute incubation period. The absorbance is read at 366, 340 or 334 nm.

Calculation

$$\Delta A/\text{min.} = \frac{A_1 - A_2}{10}$$

Measurement at 366 nm

$$\frac{\Delta A/\text{min.}}{3.3 \times 10^3} \times 10^6 \times \frac{178}{50} = \Delta A/\text{min.} \times 1080 = \text{mU/ml.}$$

Measurement at 340 nm

$$\frac{\Delta A/\text{min.}}{6.2 \times 10^3} \times 10^6 \times \frac{178}{50} = \Delta A/\text{min.} \times 572 = \text{mU/ml.}$$

Measurement at 344 nm

$$\frac{\Delta A/\text{min.}}{6.0 \times 10^3} \times 10^6 \times \frac{178}{50} = \Delta A/\text{min.} \times 592 = \text{mU/ml.}$$

With pipet volumes different from those prescribed, the factors must be recalculated (general formula on page 44).

Remarks

CPK is a sulfhydryl enzyme and is rapidly inactivated in serum. The activity in normal serum is 0–1 mU/ml, even when determined in freshly drawn blood. Elevated activity in pathological sera decreases steadily and measurements should be made as soon as possible.

G. Forster (Schweiz. Med. Wochschr. **97**, 329 [1967]) reported on the activation of CPK in serum with Cleland's reagent (dithiothreitol, DTT; Calbiochem). Reactivation is possible even in sera which were kept at room temperature for several days.

For the above method the following procedure with DTT is recommended: Cleland's reagent: 18×10^{-3}M DTT. Dissolve 27.8 mg dithiothreitol in 10 ml redistilled water.

Pipet into each of two 10-mm microcuvettes (enzyme sample and blank)

30 μl serum
20 μl DTT
35 μl glycine buffer (A)
3 μl LDH/PK (B)

and proceed as above. The calculation factors change according to the reduced amount of serum (but constant total volume).

$$366 \text{ nm } \Delta A/\text{min.} \times 1800 = \text{mU/ml serum}$$

$$340 \text{ nm } \Delta A/\text{min.} \times 953 = \text{mU/ml serum}$$

$$334 \text{ nm } \Delta A/\text{min.} \times 987 = \text{mU/ml serum}$$

Normal serum values:

without activation: 0–1 mU/ml
with Cleland's reagent: up to 7 mU/ml

Chapter 7

Enzyme Assays in Tissue Samples

The introduction of percutaneous needle biopsy has provided the opportunity to study enzymes in living tissue. The size of the tissue specimens thus obtained is between 10 and 35 mg. About 1/3 of the specimens is needed for histology. Micromethods are essential for enzyme analysis of the remaining tissue.

PREPARATION OF HOMOGENATES AND EXTRACTS

After removing it from the needle, the tissue sample is weighed immediately. Since water evaporates quickly from small pieces of tissue, weighing is repeated several times at 1 minute intervals. The weight is plotted over the time on graph paper, and the actual fresh weight is obtained by extrapolation to time zero.

The sample is homogenized with ice cooling in 0.15N NaCl, pH 7.2, or a suitable buffer, with a Potter Elvejhem all-glass homogenizer or with a Polytron PT 10*. Extracts are prepared by centrifuging at 18 000 g and +2°C.

* The Williams Polytron (Brinkmann Instruments) is a kinematic high-frequency sonic and ultrasonic homogenizer.

For the fractionated extraction and separation of enzymes in the cytoplasmic compartment (C-compartment) from the enzymes in the mitochondrial compartment (M-compartment), the following technique is recommended (E. Schmidt, and F. W. Schmidt, Enzymol. Biol. Clin. **2**, 201 [1962/63]):

C-Compartment

The tissue is homogenized in a solution containing 0.25M sucrose and 2.6 mM EDTA, pH 7.2, with a Teflon-glass homogenizer for 30 seconds (ice cooling). The homogenate is centrifuged immediately at 18 000 g and +2°C. The supernatant is used for analysis.

M-Compartment

The sediment is washed twice with sucrose-EDTA solution and then homogenized in 0.05M triethanolamine buffer, pH 7.2, with a Polytron PT 10 (ice-salt-cooling) for 4 × $\frac{1}{2}$ minute with approximately $\frac{1}{2}$ minute pauses. The homogenate is allowed to stand for 30 minutes at room temperature and is then centrifuged at 18 000 g and +2°C. The supernatant is used for analysis.

GENERAL REMARKS ON ENZYME ASSAYS IN HOMOGENATES

Enzyme assays in clear extracts with the optical test need no further commentary. Occasionally, however, measurements must be made in homogenates, and turbidity or opalescence may lead to high self-absorption by the homogenate. To compensate, an equal amount of homogenate is added to a blank containing only buffer. If it is impossible to adjust the photometer to 100% transmittance (absorbance = 0) with the homogenate blank in the light path, then the following practice is recommended. Prepare reagent mixtures in five to six micro test tubes. Then add homogenate to tube 1, mix and immediately centrifuge at about 15 000 g for 30 seconds, stop the centrifuge quickly, transfer the supernatant into a microcuvette and read absorbance (A at time 0 minutes). Not more than 1 minute should elapse in this operation. A microcentrifuge which reaches full speed in a few seconds (page 15) should be available. Then add homogenate to the remaining test tubes in suitable and exactly timed intervals (stopwatch) and incubate. At 1 to 2 minute intervals centrifuge one test tube at a time and read absorbance. Extend intervals to 3 to 5 minutes when activity is low. The change in absorbance (ΔA) should not exceed 0.03 per minute.

Dilute very active homogenates. Plot absorbance over time on graph paper and read ΔA/min. from the straight segment of the curve (example on page 41). If only a little homogenate is available, prepare only two test tubes and read at 0 minutes and 5 or 10 minutes. ΔA/5 min. should not exceed 0.100

Methods

Methods for enzyme tests in tissues have not yet been standardized. Optimum assay conditions—pH, buffer, substrate and coenzyme concentrations, etc.—may vary from organ to organ for the same enzyme and therefore must be established if quantitative comparisons are to be made. An exact record of the assay conditions should always be included in publications in order to enable comparisons. Unfortunately such details are not always presented.

The following methods were described in chapter 6. Aldolase, page 132; malate dehydrogenase, page 129; glutamate dehydrogenase, page 139; glutamate oxaloacetate transaminase, page 135; glutamate pyruvate transaminase, page 137; isocitrate dehydrogenase, page 141; lactate dehydrogenase, page 143; 1-phosphofructaldolase; page 145; phosphohexose isomerase, page 147; sorbitol dehydrogenase, page 149; alkaline phosphatase, page 161; leucine aminopeptidase, page 153; creatine phosphokinase, page 165.

By substituting homogenate or extract for serum, these procedures can be applied to enzyme studies in tissues. Whether or not the sample volume will differ from the serum volume indicated in the tests will depend on the activity of the enzyme to be measured and the concentration of a homogenate. Any difference in volume is compensated for by varying the buffer volume. Additional methods for enzyme assays in tissue homogenates or extracts are described below.

GLUCOSE-6-PHOSPHATE DEHYDROGENASE (G-6-PDH)

Literature: Glock, G. E., and P. McLean, Biochem. J. **55**, 400 (1953): micromodification: Borner, K., and H. Mattenheimer, Biochim. Biophys. Acta **34**, 592 (1959).

Principle

Glucose-6-phosphate dehydrogenase (G-6-PDH) catalyzes the reaction

$$\text{glucose-6-ph} + NADP^+ + H_2O \rightleftharpoons \text{6-phosphogluconate} + NADPH + H^+ \quad (1)$$

6-Phosphogluconate is further converted according to reaction (2) by 6-phosphogluconate dehydrogenase (6-PGDH), which is present in most organs, especially liver.

$$\text{6-phosphogluconate} + NADP^+ \rightleftharpoons \text{ribulose-5-ph} + CO_2 + NADPH + H^+ \quad (2)$$

If the activity of G-6-PDH is to be determined by measuring the rate of NADP reduction, reaction (2) must be taken into account by one of two possibilities:

(a) Measurement of the overall reduction of NADP with glucose-6-ph as substrate, and in a second assay the reduction of NADP with 6-phosphogluconate as substrate according to (2). The difference equals the NADP reduction by reaction (1).

(b) Addition of excess 6-PGDH so that 6-phosphogluconate generated in reaction (1) is converted quantitatively into ribulose-5-ph. Exactly one-half of the NADP reduction then accounts for the activity of G-6-PDH.

We prefer the measurement of G-6-PDH according to (b).

Reagents

A. *Tris buffer* 0.1M, pH 8.0

B. *$MgCl_2$* 0.3M, in redistilled water

C. *Glucose-6-phosphate* (disodium salt) 0.025M, in redistilled water

D. *NADP* 2×10^{-3}M, in redistilled water

E. *6-Phosphogluconate dehydrogenase* (6-PGDH): dissolved in Tris buffer (A). The concentration depends on the activity of the particular sample. With 6-PGDH from Sigma, prepare solution with 2 mg/ml. To determine the activity of the 6-PGDH preparation, use 6-phosphogluconate instead of glucose-6-phosphate in the assay mixture described below and replace tissue extract with buffer. The activity should be equal to an absorbance change of 0.2–0.3 per minute.

Procedure

Pipet into a 10-mm microcuvette

	200 μl buffer (A)
	10 μl $MgCl_2$ (B)
	20 μl NADP (D)
	50 μl tissue extract
	10 μl 6-PGDH (E)
Mix with polyethylene stirrer and read absorbance at 366 or 340 nm then add	
	10 μl substrate (C)
	300 μl total volume

Mix and read absorbance at one minute intervals for about 5 minutes. With ΔA exceeding 0.03/min., use less extract in assay and compensate volume with Tris buffer. Incubation temperature: 25°C. If homogenate is used instead of tissue extract, follow suggestions on page 170.

Calculation

ΔA/min. is obtained graphically (see page 41) or by calculating the mean.

Measurement at 366 nm:

$$\frac{\Delta A}{3.3 \times 10^3} \times 10^6 \times \frac{\text{total assay volume}}{\text{sample volume}} \times 0.5 =$$

$$\text{m}\mu\text{moles/min.} \times \text{ml homogenate} = \text{mU/ml homogenate}$$

With the fresh or dry weight known, the activity can be expressed in mU or U per g tissue.

GLYCEROLPHOSPHATE DEHYDROGENASE (GDH)

Literature: Beisenherz, G., T. Bücher, and K. H. Garbade, in S. P. Colowick and N. O. Kaplan, Methods in Enzymology Vol. **1**, 391 (1955).

Principle

Glycerolphosphate dehydrogenase catalyzes the reaction

$$\text{Dihydroxyacetone phosphate} + \text{NADH} + \text{H}^+ \rightleftharpoons \text{glycerol-3-phosphate} + \text{NAD}^+$$

NADH is oxidized in equimolar quantities and the rate of the oxidation is a measure of the enzyme activity.

Reagents

A. *Triethanolamine buffer* 0.06M, pH 7.5

B. *NADH* 5.4×10^{-3}M: dissolved in redistilled water or buffer (A)

C. *Dihydroxyacetone phosphate* (DAP) 3.0×10^{-3}M: dissolve the dicyclohexylammonium salt of DAP dimethylketal (mol. wt. 432.5) in redistilled water.

Procedure

Pipet into a 10-mm microcuvette	
	230 μl buffer (A)
	10 μl NADH (B)
	50 μl tissue extract
Mix with polyethylene stirrer and read absorbance at 366 or 340 nm. Wait until edogenous substrates in tissue extract have reacted with consumption of NADH. When no further decrease in absorbance occurs, add	
	10 μl substrate (C)
	300 μl total volume

Mix with polyethylene stirrer and read absorbance at 1 minute intervals for about 5 minutes. If ΔA exceeds 0.03/min., use less extract in assay and compensate volume with buffer. Incubation temperature: 25°C.

If homogenate is used instead of tissue extract, follow the suggestions on page 170.

Calculation

ΔA/min. is obtained graphically (see page 41) or by calculating the mean.

Measurement at 366 nm:

$$\frac{\Delta A}{3.3 \times 10^3} \times 10^6 \times \frac{\text{total assay volume}}{\text{sample volume}} =$$

$$\text{m}\mu\text{moles/min.} \times \text{ml homogenate} = \text{mU/ml homogenate}$$

With the fresh or dry weight known, the activity can be expressed in mU or U per g tissue.

PHOSPHOGLYCERATE KINASE (PGK)

Literature: Bücher, T., in S. P. Colowick and N. O. Kaplan, Methods in Enzymology Vol. **1**, 415 (1955); micromodification: Borner, K., and H. Mattenheimer, Biochim. Biophys. Acta **34**, 592 (1959).

Principle

Phosphoglycerate kinase (PGK) catalyzes the reaction

D-1,3-diphosphoglycerate + ADP ⇌ D-3-phosphoglycerate + ATP (1)

The reaction can be measured with a coupled optical test in either direction. The rate from left to right is about four times as high as in the reverse direction, but for PGK determinations in tissue extracts measurement from right to left is preferable. Diphosphoglycerate formed in (1) reacts further with added NADH and glyceraldehyde phosphate dehydrogenase (GAPDH).

$$\text{D-1,3-diphosphoglycerate} + \text{NADH} + \text{H}^+ \xrightleftharpoons{\text{(GAPDH)}} \text{glyceraldehydephosphate} + \text{phosphate} + \text{NAD}^+ \quad (2)$$

Glyceraldehyde phosphate is trapped with cysteine. NADH is oxidized in equimolar quantities and the rate of oxidation is a measure of the PGK activity.

Reagents

A. *Triethanolamine buffer* 0.075M, pH 7.5

B. *D-3-phosphoglycerate solution* 1.5×10^{-1}M: dissolve the trisodium salt (mol. wt. 252.1) or the tricyclohexylammonium salt $\times$ 3 H_2O (mol. wt. 537.6) in redistilled water.

C. *ATP solution* 9×10^{-3}M

D. *$MgSO_4$ solution* 1.5×10^{-2}M

E. *NADH solution* 5.4×10^{-3}M: in redistilled water or buffer (A)

F. *Cysteine solution* 6×10^{-1}M

G. *Glyceraldehyde phosphate dehydrogenase* (GAPDH): 4 mg/ml; commercially available as suspension in ammonium sulfate solution. Minimum activity: 25 U/mg enzyme protein.

The reproducibility of the data depends especially on the exact concentration of the substrate and the $MgSO_4$ solutions.

Procedure

Pipet into a 10-mm microcuvette

	200 μl buffer (A)
	10 μl NADH (E)
	10 μl ATP (C)
	10 μl $MgSO_4$ (D)
	10 μl cysteine (F)
	5 μl GAPDH (G)
	50 μl tissue extract
Mix with polyethylene stirrer and read absorbance at 366 or 340 nm. Wait until endogenous substrates in the extract have reacted with consumption of NADH. When no further decrease in absorbance occurs, add	
	10 μl substrate (B)
	305 μl total volume

Mix and read absorbance at one minute intervals for about five minutes. If ΔA exceeds 0.03/min., use less extract in assay and compensate volume with buffer. Incubation temperature: 25°C. If homogenate is used instead of tissue extract, follow suggestions on page 170.

Calculation

ΔA/min. is obtained graphically (see page 41) or by calculating the mean.

Measurement at 366 nm:

$$\frac{\Delta A}{3.3 \times 10^3} \times 10^6 \times \frac{\text{total assay volume}}{\text{sample volume}} =$$

$$\text{m}\mu\text{moles/min.} \times \text{ml homogenate} = \text{mU/ml homogenate}$$

With the fresh or dry weight known, the activity can be expressed in mU or U per g tissue.

PYRUVATE KINASE (PK)

Literature: Bücher, T., and G. Pfleiderer, in S. P. Colowick and N. O. Kaplan, Methods of Enzymology Vol. **1**, 435 (1955); micromodification: Borner, K., and H. Mattenheimer, Biochim. Biophys. Acta **34**, 592 (1959).

Principle

Pyruvate kinase (PK) catalyzes the reaction

$$\text{ADP} + \text{phosphoenol pyruvate} \rightleftharpoons \text{ATP} + \text{pyruvate}$$

Pyruvate is reduced to lactate in a coupled reaction with NADH and lactate dehydrogenase (LDH)

$$\text{Pyruvate} + \text{NADH} + \text{H}^+ \xrightleftharpoons{\text{(LDH)}} \text{lactate} + \text{NAD}^+$$

NADH is oxidized in equimolar amounts and the rate of oxidation is a measure of the PK activity.

Reagents

A. *Triethanolamine buffer* 0.075M, pH 7.5

B. *ADP solution* 7×10^{-3}M

C. *Phosphoenol pyruvate (PEP) solution* 2.3×10^{-2}M: dissolve the tricyclohexylammonium salt (mol. wt. 465.6) in redistilled water.

D. *$MgSO_4$-KCl solution* 2.4×10^{-1}M, 2.25M, respectively.

E. *NADH solution* 5.4×10^{-3}M: in redistilled water or in buffer (A).

F. *Lactate dehydrogenase*: 0.5 mg/ml.
Commercially available as suspension in ammonium sulfate solution. Minimum activity: 300 U/mg enzyme protein.

Procedure

Pipet into a 10-mm microcuvette

210 μl	buffer	(A)
10 μl	ADP	(B)
10 μl	PEP	(C)
10 μl	$MgSO_4$/KCl	(D)
10 μl	NADH	(E)
2 μl	LDH	(F)

Mix with polyethylene stirrer and read absorbance at 366 or 340 nm. Traces of pyruvate in PEP react with NADH and LDH. When no further decrease in absorbance occurs, add

50 μl tissue extract

302 μl total volume

Mix and read absorbance at 1 minute intervals for about 5 minutes. If ΔA exceeds 0.03/min., use less extract in assay and compensate volume with buffer. Incubation temperature: 25°C. If homogenate is used instead of tissue extract follow suggestions on page 170.

Calculation

ΔA/min. is obtained graphically (see page 41) or by calculating the mean.

Measurement at 366 nm:

$$\frac{\Delta A}{3.3 \times 10^3} \times 10^6 \times \frac{\text{total assay volume}}{\text{sample volume}} =$$

$$\text{m}\mu\text{moles/min.} \times \text{ml homogenate} = \text{mU/ml homogenate}$$

With the fresh or dry weight known, the activity can be expressed in mU or U per g tissue.

TRIOSEPHOSPHATE ISOMERASE (TIM)

Literature: Beisenherz, G., in S. P. Colowick and N. O. Kaplan, Methods in Enzymology Vol. **1**, 387 (1955).

Principle

Triosephosphate isomerase (TIM) catalyzes the reaction

D-glyceraldehyde-3-phosphate $\rightleftharpoons$ dihydroxyacetone phosphate

In a coupled indicator reaction with NADH and glycerol-3-phosphate dehydrogenase (GDH), dihydroxyacetone phosphate is reduced to glycerol-3-phosphate.

dihydroxyacetone phosphate + NADH + H^+ $\rightleftharpoons$
glycerol-3-phosphate + NAD^+

NADH is oxidized in equimolar amounts and the rate of oxidation is a measure of the TIM activity.

Reagents

A. *Triethanolamine buffer* 0.03M, pH 7.9

B. *NADH solution* 5.4×10^{-3} M: dissolved in redistilled water or in buffer (A)

C. DL-*glyceraldehyde-3-phosphate* 9×10^{-3}M (= 4.5×10^{-3}M D-form)

D. *Glycerol-3-phosphate dehydrogenase* (GDH): 1 mg/ml. Commercially available as suspension in ammonium sulfate solution. Minimum activity: 70 U/mg enzyme protein.

Procedure

Pipet into a *20*-mm microcuvette

460 μl buffer (A)
20 μl NADH (B)
4 μl GDH (D)
100 μl tissue extract

Mix with polyethylene stirrer and read absorbance at 366 or 340 nm. Wait until endogenous substrates in the extract have reacted with consumption of NADH. When no further decrease in absorbance occurs, add

	20 μl substrate (C)
	604 μl total volume

Mix with polyethylene stirrer and read absorbance at 1 minute intervals for 5–10 minutes. If ΔA exceeds 0.03/min., use less extract in assay and compensate volume with buffer. Incubation temperature: 25°C. If homogenate is used instead of tissue extract follow suggestions on page 170.

Calculation

ΔA/min. is obtained graphically (see page 41) or by calculating the mean.

Measurement at 366 nm

$$\frac{\Delta A}{3.3 \times 10^3} \times 10^6 \times \frac{\text{total assay volume}}{\text{sample volume}} \times 0.5 =$$
$$\text{m}\mu\text{moles/min.} \times \text{ml homogenate} = \text{mU/ml homogenate}$$

With the fresh or dry weight known, the activity can be expressed in mU or U per g tissue.

GLUTAMINASES

Literature: Mattenheimer, H., and H. DeBruin, Enzymol. Biol. Clin. **4**, 65 (1964).

Principle

At least three glutaminases are present in tissue from man and mammals. Glutaminase I is activated by phosphate ions and hydrolyzes glutamine to glutamate and NH_3; glutaminase II is activated by 2-oxo-acids and catalyzes two steps

$$\text{glutamine} + \text{2-oxo-acid} \longrightarrow \text{2-oxo-glutaramate} + \text{amino acid} \quad (1)$$

$$\text{2-oxo-glutaramate} \longrightarrow \text{2-oxo-glutarate} + NH_3 \quad (2)$$

The non-activated glutaminase hydrolyzes glutamine to glutamate and NH_3 in the absence of phosphate or a 2-oxo-acid. Glutaminase activity is determined by titration of NH_3 released and separated from the reaction mixture by microdiffusion. Enzyme reaction, diffusion and titration are performed in one micro test tube.

Reagents

A. *Tris buffer* 0.2M, pH 9.0

B. *Na_2HPO_4 solution,* 1.0M, adjusted to pH 8.75 with NaH_2PO_4

C. *Na-pyruvate,* 0.5M, adjusted to pH 8.75 with NaOH

D. *Glutamine* 0.12M, adjusted to pH 8.75 with NaOH: prepared fresh daily.

E. *K_2CO_3*, saturated solution

F. *Boric acid* 2%

G. *Indicator solution*: 3 volumes of 0.1% Bromocresol Green in 95% ethanol, mixed with 1 volume 0.2% Methyl Red in 95% ethanol.

H. *Boric acid indicator solution*: to 5 ml (F) add 60 μl (G)

I. *H_2SO_4*: 0.020N

K. *Buffer-activator-solution for glutaminase I:* mix equal volumes of (A) and (B).

L. *Buffer-activator-solution for glutaminase II:* mix equal volumes of (A) and (C).

M. *Buffer for nonactivated glutaminase:* mix equal volumes of (A) with redistilled water.

Tissue homogenates

Extremely low glutaminase activities are found in human tissue obtained at autopsy. It is therefore essential to determine glutaminase activity in tissue obtained by needle or surgical biopsy and to carry out the assay immediately thereafter. Animal tissues have to be obtained by surgery or immediately after the animal was sacrificed. 10% (w/v) tissue homogenates are prepared in redistilled water with a Potter-Elvejhem homogenizer. Homogenization with blendor homogenizers destroys the activity almost completely.

The 10% homogenates are used for the measurement of glutaminase II and nonactivated glutaminase. A 1:2 to 1:4 dilution is recommended for glutaminase I. If the calculations are to be based on fresh weight, the tissue is weighed on a microbalance (*e.g.*, Cahn electrobalance, see notes for weighing on page 169). For calculation based on dry weight, an aliquot of the homogenate is dried at 110°C.

Equipment

Constriction pipets: 5 μl, 10 μl, 20 μl and a double constriction pipet 40 μl (see Figure 31); micro test tubes: 30 × 4 mm internally coated with silicone (see page 34). The freshly coated tubes are heated at 150°C for at least 2 hours.

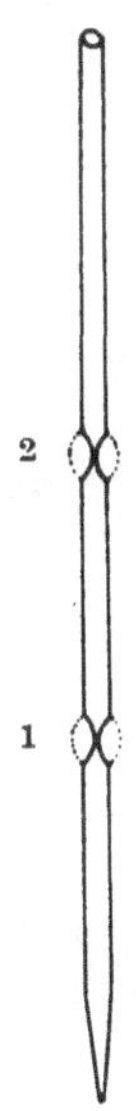

Figure 31. Polyethylene double-constriction pipet, for pipetting the boric acid seal. Volume between 1 and 2 ~ 40 μl.

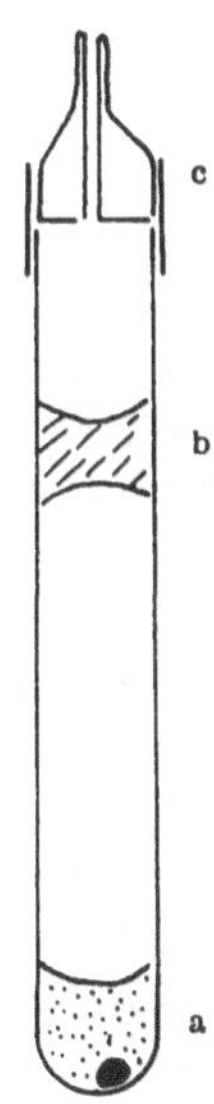

Figure 32. Microdiffusion of NH_3. Micro test tube (4 × 30 mm).
a. incubation mixture with mixer (flea).
b. boric acid seal.
c. stopper, made from rubber tubing with drawn out glass tubing.

Magnetic stirrers ("fleas"): see page 24; rotator: see Figure 33; strong magnet to operate the "fleas."

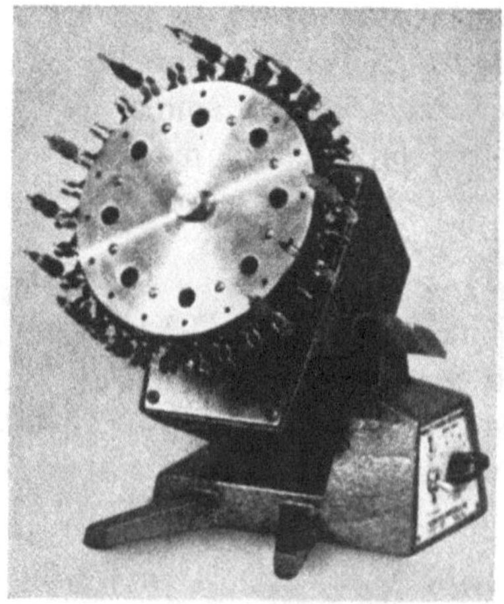

Figure 33. Rotator with micro test tubes (as in Figure 32).

Procedure

Place test tubes in ice bath and add one flea to each. Pipet into test tubes

10 μl buffered activator solution (K) or (L) or (M)
10 μl glutamine (D)
5 μl homogenate

Mixing is achieved by moving the fleas with the magnet. The tubes are capped with Parafilm and incubated at 37°C. At the end of the incubation period, 30 minutes for glutaminase I and 60 minutes for the other glutaminases, the test tubes are returned to the ice bath.

NH_3 determination

To each test tube add 20 μl of K_2CO_3 solution (E) and seal with boric acid (H), using the double constriction pipet. The following technique is recommended to avoid a loss of NH_3: hold the test tube horizontally and place the carbonate solution on the test tube wall about 2 mm above the surface of the incubation medium. Under no circumstances must the pipet touch the test tube wall higher up; otherwise alkali could contaminate the boric acid seal. Still holding the test tube in the horizontal position form a seal with the boric acid in the upper third of the test tube. Fill the double constriction pipet to constriction 2 (see Figure 31) with boric acid (H). Set the tip of the pipet on the wall of the test tube where the seal is to be formed, and slowly deliver the fluid by applying slight pressure through the mouth tube. During delivery of the fluid rotate the test tube slowly around its axis to form the seal. The pipet is emptied to constriction 1 after the seal has formed.

The next step is to mix the carbonate solution into the incubation medium with the magnetic stirrer. To avoid evaporation of sealing fluid, the test tubes are capped with rubber caps with a capillary opening (see Figure 32). The test tubes are then rotated for 2 hours at room temperature. The rotator is set at an angle so that the fleas accomplish stirring by their gravity.

For the titration one test tube is placed in the vibrator holder (see Figure 34) beside a test tube filled with boric acid (H). The tip of the polyethylene tube which is connected to the tip of the titrator (has to be filled bubble-free) is lowered into the seal. To increase the mixing effect gradually, the vibrator must be connected to a powerstat; otherwise the

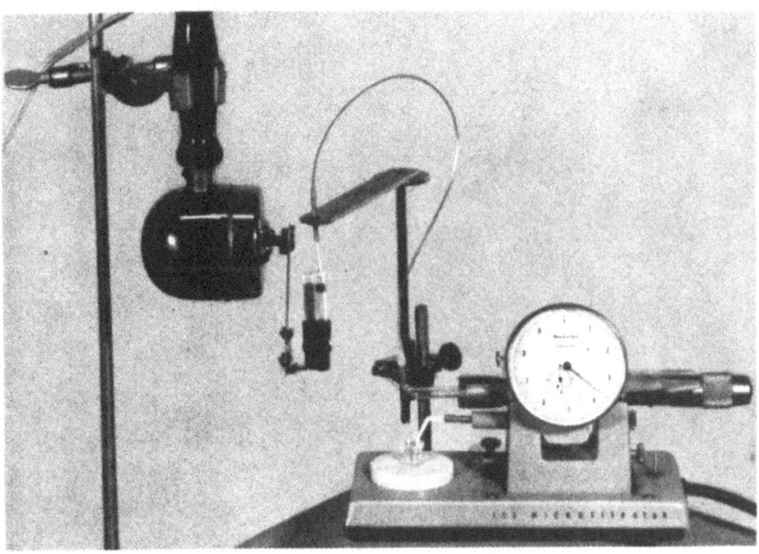

Figure 34. Microtitration assembly for the determination of NH_3, vibrator with holder for micro test tubes. Adjustable support to dip the polyethylene tubing into the boric acid seal. Beckman-Spinco 153 Microtitrator. One revolution of the hand = 1.00 μl.

seal will break up. The seal is then titrated with 0.020N H_2SO_4 (I). The color change from green to red is easy to observe and can best be seen against a background of diffuse white light.

Calculation

1 μl 0.020N H_2SO_4 = 20 mμmoles NH_3
V = volume of H_2SO_4 in μl
t = incubation time in minutes
G = weight of tissue in test tube in μg (dry weight or wet weight)

$$\frac{V \times 20 \times 10^{-3}}{t \times G \times 10^{-6}} = \mu\text{moles } NH_3/\text{g} \times \text{min.}$$

Blanks

Prepare two or three blanks with each of the buffer activator solutions (K, L, and M) and add water instead of homogenate. A slight but measurable hydrolysis of glutamine occurs in alkaline solutions, particularly in the presence of phosphate (glutaminase I). The blank value is subtracted.

$$V = V_{\text{sample}} - V_{\text{blank}}$$

Homogenate blanks (without glutamine) should be checked for each tissue. In the author's experience they can be omitted for kidney and liver.

Chapter 8

Determination of Enzymes with Ultramicromethods

Literature: Lowry, O. H., J. Histochem. Cytochem. **1**, 420 (1953); Lowry, O. H., N. R. Roberts, K. Y. Leiner, M. L. Wu, and A. L. Farr, J. Biol. Chem. **207**, 1 (1954); Lowry, O. H., N. R. Roberts, M. L. Wu, W. S. Hixon, and E. J. Crawford, J. Biol. Chem. **207**, 19 (1954); Lowry, O. H., N. R. Roberts, K. Y. Leiner, M. L. Wu, A. L. Farr, and R. W. Albers, J. Biol. Chem. **207**, 39 (1954); Strominger, J. L., and O. H. Lowry, J. Biol. Chem. **213**, 635 (1955); Robins, E., N. R. Roberts, K. M. Eydt, O. H. Lowry, and D. E. Smith, J. Biol. Chem. **218**, 897 (1955); Lowry, O. H., N. R. Roberts, and C. Lewis, J. Biol Chem. **220**, 879 (1956); Lowry, O. H., N. R. Roberts, and M. W. Chang, J. Biol. Chem. **222**, 97 (1956); Burch, H. B., O. H. Lowry, A. M. Padilla, and A. M. Combs, J. Biol. Chem. **223**, 29 (1956); Buell, M. V., O. H. Lowry, N. R. Roberts, M. W. Chang, and J. I. Kapphahn, J. Biol. Chem. **232**, 979 (1958); Lowry, O. H., Harvey Lectures, series 58, 1962/63, page 1.

This chapter describes ultramicro procedures, published mainly by O. H. Lowry and his associates, for a quantitative determination of enzyme activity in minute amountes of frozen-dried tissue samples (order of magnitude 10^{-3} μg) or in less than 1 μl tissue homogenate or body fluids.

Similar to the optical test, NAD (NADP)-dependent enzyme reactions are measured by the rate of oxidation or reduction of the pyridine nucleotides. But instead of reading the absorbance at 340 nm or 366 nm, NAD (NADP) is converted chemically into a fluorescent compound by treatment with alkali. The sensitivity is thereby increased about 1000-fold, and pyridine nucleotides can be measured in concentrations as low as 10^{-8}M.

The methods, originally designed by Lowry to measure enzymes in brain tissue and the retina, were adapted in our laboratory to determine enzyme activity in the nephron (B. S. L. Bonting *et al.*, Science **127**, 1343 [1958]). The assay conditions—pH optima, substrate and coenzyme concentrations, etc.—delineated in the following procedures are those for kidney tissue and must be verified for applicability to other tissues and body fluids.

PRELIMINARY REMARKS

In work with frozen-dried tissue, the enzyme activity is preferably expressed per unit dry weight. The specimens are weighed on quartz-fiber balances with sensitivities ranging from less than 1 to about 10 mμg. The construction of quartz-fiber balances and other equipment for ultramicro analysis, especially for handling ultramicro samples, is described in detail in Lowry's publications.

The incubation volume ranges from about 1 to 10 μl. To avoid evaporation, the surface area of the fluid must be kept at a minimum. It is therefore necessary to use micro test tubes with an inside diameter of 3 mm and a length of about 50 mm (page 27). The test tubes are capped with Parafilm. The small diameter requires constriction pipets with long tips, which are not commercially available but have to be made in the laboratory. Polyethylene constriction pipets are easy to make and are highly recommended for ultramicro analysis (page 17).

Mixing of small amounts of fluid is best achieved by vibration (page 26). if a frozen-dried tissue specimen has been added to the incubation medium, mixing should be avoided because the specimen might be projected from the fluid and adhere to the test tube wall.

The Farrand Model A Fluorometer (Farrand Optical Company, Bronx, New York) is recommended for fluorometric estimations. Measurements can be made directly in 10 × 75-mm test tubes with a minimum volume of 1 ml. A special adapter permits the use of smaller test tubes with a considerable volume reduction. However, any other fluorometer of sufficient sensitivity is also satisfactory.

All assay mixtures contain bovine serum albumin (0.05%) to avoid inactivation of enzymes by denaturation in high dilutions, and nicotinamide (0.02M) to inhibit nucleotidases.

PRINCIPLE OF FLUOROMETRIC DETERMINATION OF PYRIDINE NUCLEOTIDES

a. Determination of NAD (NADP)

Hydrochloric acid is added to the sample to give a concentration of 0.2N. NADH (NADPH) is thus destroyed within 30 seconds at room temperature. NaOH is then added to a final concentration of 6N and the sample is allowed to stand for 30 minutes at 37°C or 60 minutes at room temperature. A fluorescent compound is formed in direct proportion to the concentration of NAD (NADP). After at least 5-fold dilution with water, fluorescence is measured with a Corning primary filter #5860 (isolates the Hg line at 365 nm) and Corning secondary filters #4308, 5562, 3387 (the combination has the maximal transmission at 470 nm). Quinine solutions in 0.1N H_2SO_4 serve as working standards (0.005–5 μg/ml).

b. Determination of NADH (NADPH)

The sample is brought to 0.04N in NaOH and incubated for 15 minutes at 60°C or for 2 hours at 37°C. In the weakly alkaline solution NAD (NADP) is degraded to a nonfluorescing compound. In the next step NADH (NADPH) is oxidized with H_2O_2 to NAD (NADP) and converted into the fluorescent compound with 6N NaOH.

STANDARDIZATION OF NAD SOLUTIONS

Principle

NAD is reduced to NADH by ethanol and alcohol dehydrogenase

$$\text{ethanol} + \text{NAD}^+ \rightleftharpoons \text{acetaldehyde} + \text{NADH} + \text{H}^+$$

Acetaldehyde is trapped with semicarbazide and NADH is determined photometrically at 340 nm or 366 nm.

Reagents

A. *NAD solution:* concentration up to about 10×10^{-3}M
B. *Ethanol-pyrophosphate solution:* to 3 ml 99% ethanol add 97 ml of a solution containing 0.075M $Na_4P_2O_7$, 0.075 M semicarbazide-HCl, 0.022M glycine, pH adjusted to 8.7 with 2N NaOH.
C. *Alcohol dehydrogenase:* commercial enzyme suspension

Procedure

Pipet into a 10-mm macrocuvette		
	3 ml ethanol solution	(B)
	35 μl NAD solution	(A)
Mix with plastic rod and read absorbance (= A_1). Then mix in	10 μl enzyme	(C)
	3.045 ml total volume	

The absorbance increases; end point = A_2.

Calculation

$$A_2 - A_1 = \Delta A$$

Measurement at 366 nm:

$$\text{mmoles NAD/liter} = \frac{3045}{35} \times \frac{\Delta A}{3.30}$$

Measurement at 340 nm:

$$= \frac{3045}{35} \times \frac{\Delta A}{6.20}$$

STANDARDIZATION OF NADP SOLUTIONS

Principle

In the presence of glucose-6-phosphate NADP is reduced to NADPH by glucose-6-phosphate dehydrogenase

$$\text{glucose-6-phosphate} + H_2O + NADP^+ \rightleftharpoons \text{6-phosphogluconate} + NADPH + H^+$$

NADPH is determined photometrically at 340 or 366 nm.

Reagents

A. *Tris buffer* 0.05M, pH 8.0
B. *$MgCl_2$ solution* 0.3M
C. *Glucose-6-phosphate* 2.5×10^{-2}M
D. *Glucose-6-phosphate dehydrogenase:* commercial enzyme suspension
E. *NADP solution:* concentration up to about 10×10^{-3}M

Procedure

Pipet into a 10-mm macrocuvette

	2.8 ml	buffer	(A)
	100 μl	$MgCl_2$	(B)
	100 μl	G-6-P	(C)
	35 μl	NADP solution	(E)
Mix with plastic rod and read absorbance (= A_1). Then mix in			
	20 μl	enzyme	(D)
	3.055 ml	total volume.	

The absorbance increases; end point = A_2.

Calculation

$A_2 - A_1 = \Delta A$

Measurement at 366 nm:

$$\text{mmoles NADP/liter} = \frac{3055}{35} \times \frac{\Delta A}{3.3}$$

Measurement at 340 nm:

$$= \frac{3055}{35} \times \frac{\Delta A}{6.2}$$

STANDARDIZATION OF NADH (NADPH) SOLUTIONS

Principle

The absorbance of a NADH (NADPH) solution is read at 340 or 366 nm before and after destruction of the pyridine nucleotides with HCl. The concentration is calculated from the absorbance difference.

Reagents

A. *Tris buffer* 0.05M, pH 8.0

B. *HCl* approximately 10N

C. *NADH (NADPH) solution*: concentration up to 10×10^{-3}M

Procedure

Pipet into a 10-mm macrocuvette

	1.95 ml buffer	(A)
	50 µl NADH (NADPH) solution	(C)

Mix with plastic rod and read absorbance (= A_1). Then mix in

	40 µl HCl	(B)

The absorbance decreases; end point = A_2.

Calculation

$A_1 - A_2 = \Delta A$

Measurement at 366 nm:

$$\text{mmoles NADH (NADPH)/liter} = \frac{2000}{50} \times \frac{\Delta A}{3.3}$$

Measurement at 340 nm:

$$= \frac{2000}{50} \times \frac{\Delta A}{6.2}$$

The volume of HCl can be neglected in the calculation.

GLUTAMATE OXALOACETATE TRANSAMINASE (GOT)

Principle

GOT catalyzes the reaction

$$\text{glutamate} + \text{oxaloacetate} \rightleftharpoons \text{aspartate} + \text{2-oxoglutarate}$$

In the reaction, proceeding from right to left, the rate of formation of oxaloacetate is measured with an indicator reaction catalyzed by malate dehydrogenase (MDH).

$$\text{oxaloacetate} + \text{NADH} + H^+ \xrightleftharpoons{\text{(MDH)}} \text{malate} + \text{NAD}^+$$

NAD^+ is formed in stoichiometric amounts and is determined fluorometrically after destruction of excess NADH.

Reagents

A. *Stock solution:*
- 2.0 ml 0.2M Tris buffer, pH 7.7
- 2.5 ml 0.1M L-aspartate solution, neutralized
- 0.2 ml 0.5M nicotinamide solution
- 0.5 ml 0.1M 2 oxoglutarate solution, neutralized
- 0.05 ml 10% bovine serum albumin solution

Stored frozen, the solution is stable for about two weeks.

B. *Incubation medium* (to be prepared every day)
- 1.0 ml stock solution
- 0.010 ml pyridoxal phosphate solution (1 mg/ml)
- 0.100 ml 3×10^{-2}M NADH solution
- 0.010 ml MDH (commercial suspension, see page 135).

C. *NAD standard*
- 10 μl 1×10^{-2}M NAD solution + 100 μl incubation medium.

D. *HCl* 0.3N

E. *NaOH* 7N

Procedure

a. Enzyme assay

(1) Depending on enzyme activity, incubate 0.01–0.1 μg frozen-dried tissue samples or 0.1–1.0 μl homogenate in 3 × 50-mm micro test tubes with 5 μl incubation medium (B). Incubation time: 30–60 minutes, temperature: 37°C.

(2) Stop enzyme reaction with 10 μl HCl (D) and mix with vibrator.

(3) Transfer 10 μl of the acid mixture into a fluorometer test tube, add 100 μl NaOH (E), mix with vibrator and incubate for 30 minutes at 37°C.

(4) Add 1.0 ml redistilled water, mix and read fluorescence against a quinine standard.

b. NAD standard: incubate 5 μl NAD standard (C) and proceed as with enxyme assay (2–4).

c. Reagent blank: incubate 5 μl incubation medium (B) and proceed as with enzyme assay (2–4).

If the enzyme activity is measured in homogenates, a corresponding volume of redistilled water is added to (b) and (c).

Calculation

Measurements are made in a fluorometer against a quinine standard (page 191). The concentration of the quinine standard should be such that a high reading with the NAD standard is achieved on the fluorometer scale. The reagent blank (c) is subtracted from (a) and (b). The calculation is based on the NAD standard. Enzyme activity is expressed in μmoles/min. × g dry weight.

GLUTAMATE PYRUVATE TRANSAMINASE (GPT)

Principle

GPT catalyzes the reaction

$$\text{glutamate} + \text{pyruvate} \rightleftharpoons \text{alanine} + \text{2-oxoglutarate}$$

In the reaction, proceeding from right to left, the rate of formation of pyruvate is measured with an indicator reaction catalyzed by lactate dehydrogenase (LDH)

$$\text{pyruvate} + \text{NADH} + H^+ \xrightleftharpoons{\text{(LDH)}} \text{lactate} + NAD^+$$

NAD^+ is formed in stoichiometric quantities and is determined fluorometrically after destruction of excess NADH.

Reagents

A. *Stock solution*:
  2.0 ml 0.2M Tris buffer, pH 7.7
  0.25 ml 0.1M 2-oxoglutarate, neutralized
  0.015 ml 10% bovine serum albumin solution
  0.1 ml 0.5M nicotinamide solution
  0.15 ml pyridoxal phosphate solution (1 mg/ml)
  Stored frozen, the solution is stable for about two weeks.

B. *Incubation medium* (to be prepared fresh every day)
  1.0 ml stock solution
  0.100 ml 3×10^{-2}M NADH solution
  0.100 ml 0.6M L-alanine solution
  0.010 ml lactate dehydrogenase (commercial suspension see page 137).

C. *NAD standard*: 10 μl 1×10^{-3}M NAD solution + 100 μl incubation medium

D. *HCl* 0.3N

E. *NaOH* 7N

Procedure

a. Enzyme assay

  (1) Depending on enzyme activity, incubate 0.01–0.1 μg frozen-dried tissue samples or 0.1–1.0 μl homogenate in 3 × 50-mm micro test tubes with 5 μl incubation medium (B). Incubation time: 30–60 minutes; temperature: 37°C.

(2) Stop enzyme reaction with 10 μl HCl (D) and mix with vibrator.

(3) Transfer 10 μl of the acid mixture into a fluorometer test tube, add 100 μl NaOH (E), mix with vibrator and incubate for 30 minutes at 37°C.

(4) Add 1.0 ml redistilled water, mix and read fluorescence against a quinine standard.

b. NAD standard: incubate 5 μl NAD standard (C) and proceed as with enzyme assay (2–4).

c. Reagent blank: incubate 5 μl incubation medium (B) and proceed as with enzyme assay (2–4). If the enzyme activity is measured in homogenates a corresponding volume of redistilled water is added to (b) and (c).

Calculation

Measurements are made in a fluorometer against a quinine standard. (page 191). The concentration of the quinine standard should be such that a high reading with the NAD standard is achieved on the fluorometer scale.

The reagent blank (c) is subtracted from (a) and (b). The calculation is based on the NAD standard. Enzyme activity is expressed in μmoles/min. × g dry weight.

LACTATE DEHYDROGENASE (LDH)

Principle

LDH catalyzes the reaction

$$\text{pyruvate} + \text{NADH} + \text{H}^+ \rightleftharpoons \text{lactate} + \text{NAD}^+$$

NAD is determined fluorometrically after destruction of excess NADH.

Reagents

A. *Stock solution:*
 4.5 ml 0.2M Tris buffer, pH 7.15
 0.250 ml 0.5M nicotinamide solution
 0.050 ml 0.1M Na-pyruvate solution
 0.025 ml 10% bovine serum albumin solution
 Stored frozen, the solution is stable for about two weeks.

B. *Incubation medium* (to be prepared every day):
 1.0 ml stock solution
 0.050 ml 2.5×10^{-2}M NADH solution

C. *NAD standard:* 4μl 1×10^{-2}M NAD solution + 100 μl incubation medium (B)

D. *HCl* 1.0N

E. *NaOH* 7N

Procedure

a. Enzyme assay
 (1) Depending on enzyme activity, incubate 0.001–0.1 μg frozen-dried tissue samples or 0.1–1.0 μl homogenate in 3 × 50-mm micro test tubes with 10 μl incubation medium (B). Incubation time: 30–60 minutes, temperature: 37°C.
 (2) Stop enzyme reaction with 2 μl HCl (D) and mix with vibrator.
 (3) Transfer 10 μl of the acid mixture into a fluorometer test tube, add 100 μl NaOH (E), mix with vibrator and incubate for 30 minutes at 37°C.
 (4) Add 1.0 ml redistilled water, mix and read fluorescence against a quinine standard.

b. NAD standard: incubate 10 μl incubation medium (C) and proceed as with enzyme assay (2–4).

c. Reagent blank: incubate 10 μl incubation medium (B) and proceed as with enzyme assay (2–4). If the enzyme activity is measured in homogenates, a corresponding volume of redistilled water is added to (b) and (c).

Calculation

Measurements are made in a fluorometer against a quinine standard (page 191). The concentration of the quinine standard should be such that a high reading with the NAD standard is achieved on the fluorometer scale. The reagent blank (c) is subtracted from the values of (a) and (b). The calculation is based on the NAD standard. Enzyme activity is expressed in μmoles/min. × g dry weight.

GLUTAMATE DEHYDROGENASE (GLDH)

Principle

GLDH catalyzes the reaction

$$\text{glutamate} + H_2O + NAD^+ \rightleftharpoons \text{2-oxoglutarate} + NH_4^+ + NADH + H^+$$

Under the experimental conditions, the equilibrium is on the side of NAD and glutamate. NAD is determined fluorometrically after destruction of excess NADH.

Reagents

A. *Stock solution*:
   4.5 ml 0.1M Tris buffer, pH 7.6
   0.125 ml 0.1M 2-oxoglutarate solution, neutralized
   0.200 ml 0.5M nicotinamide solution
   0.125 ml 3.0M ammonium sulfate solution
   0.025 ml 10% bovine serum albumin solution
   Stored frozen, the solution is stable for about 2 weeks.

B. *Incubation medium* (to be prepared fresh every day):
   1.0 ml stock solution
   0.100 ml 3×10^{-2}M NADH solution

C. *NAD standard*: 5 μl 1×10^{-2}M NAD solution + 100 μl incubation medium

D. *HCl* 0.3N

E. *NaOH* 7N

Procedure

a. Enzyme assay
   (1) Depending on enzyme activity, incubate 0.01–0.1 μg frozen-dried tissue samples or 0.1–1.0 μl homogenate in 3 × 50-mm micro test tubes with 5 μl incubation medium (B). Incubation time: 30–60 minutes; temperature: 37°C.
   (2) Stop enzyme reaction with 10 μl HCl (D) and mix with vibrator.
   (3) Transfer 10 μl of the acid mixture into a fluorometer test tube, add 100 μl NaOH (E), mix with vibrator and incubate for 30 minutes at 37°C.
   (4) Add 1.0 ml redistilled water, mix and read fluorescence against a quinine standard.

b. NAD standard: incubate 5 μl NAD standard (C) and proceed as with enzyme assay (2–4).
c. Reagent blank: incubate 5 μl incubation medium (B) and proceed as with enzyme assay (2–4). If the enzyme activity is measured in homogenates, a corresponding volume of redistilled water is added to (b) and (c).

Calculation

Measurements are made in a fluorometer against a quinine standard (page 191). The concentration of the quinine standard should be such that a high reading with the NAD standard is achieved on the fluorometer scale.

The reagent blank (c) is subtracted from the values of (a) and (b). The calculation is based on the NAD standard. Enzyme activity is expressed in μmoles/min. × g dry weight.

GLUCOSE-6-PHOSPHATE DEHYDROGENASE (G-6-PDH)

Principle

G-6-PDH catalyzes the reaction

$$\text{glucose-6-phosphate} + NADP^+ + H_2O \rightleftharpoons \text{6-phosphogluconate} + NADPH + H^+ \quad (1)$$

6-phosphogluconate is further converted according to reaction (2) by 6-phosphogluconate dehydrogenase (6-PGDH) which is present in most tissues, especially liver.

$$\text{6-phosphogluconate} + NADP^+ \rightleftharpoons \text{ribulose-5-phosphate} + CO_2 + NADPH + H^+ \quad (2)$$

If the activity of G-6-PDH is to be determined by measuring the rate of NADP reduction, reaction (2) must be taken into account. This is best be done by adding an excess of 6-PGDH to convert the 6-phosphogluconate generated in reaction (1) quantitatively to ribulose-5-phosphate. Exactly one-half of the NADP reduction accounts for the activity of G-6-PDH. To measure NADPH generated in the enzyme reactions, excess NADP is destroyed and NADPH oxidized to NADP, which is then determined fluorometrically. This procedure deviates from the method described by Lowry.

Reagents

A. *Incubation medium:*

600 μl 0.15M aminomethylpropanediol buffer, pH 8.0

50 μl 0.1M glucose-6-phosphate solution

10 μl 0.1M ethylenediaminotetraacetate (Na_4) solution

100 μl 0.1M $MgCl_2$ solution

200 μl 1×10^{-2}M NADP solution

5 μl 10% bovine serum albumin solution

35 μl 6-phosphogluconate dehydrogenase (commercial preparation, see page 172).

B. *NADPH standard solution*: 10 μl 1×10^{-2}M NADPH solution + 100 μl incubation medium (A)

C. *NaOH* 0.06N

D. *NaOH* 7.0N with 0.01% H_2O_2

Procedure

a. Enzyme assay
   (1) Depending on the enzyme activity, incubate 0.01–0.1 μg frozen-dried tissue samples or 0.1–1.0 μl homogenate in 3 × 50-mm micro test tubes with 5 μl incubation medium (A). Incubation time: 30–60 minutes; temperature: 37°C.
   (2) Stop reaction with 10 μl 0.06N NaOH (C), mix with vibrator and incubate for 15 minutes at 60°C.
   (3) Transfer 10 μl of the alkaline mixture into a fluorometer test tube, add 100 μl NaOH with H_2O_2 (D), mix with vibrator and incubate for 30 minutes at 37°C.
   (4) Add 1.0 ml redistilled water, mix and read fluorescence against a quinine standard.

b. NADPH standard: incubate 5 μl NADPH standard (B) and proceed as with enzyme assay (2–4).

c. Reagent blank: incubate 5 μl incubation medium (A) and proceed as with enzyme assay (2–4). If the enzyme activity is measured in homogenates, a corresponding volume of redistilled water is added to (b) and (c).

Calculation

Measurements are made in a fluorometer against a quinine standard (page 191). The concentration of the quinine standard should be such that a high reading with the NAD standard is achieved on the fluorometer scale.

The reagent blank (c) is subtracted from (a) and (b). The calculation is based on the NADH standard. Enzyme activity is expressed in μmoles/min. × g dry weight.

ATP PHOSPHOHYDROLASE (ATPase)

Principle

ATPase hydrolyzes adenosine triphosphate (ATP) to adenosine diphosphate (ADP) and inorganic phosphate. Phosphate is determined colorimetrically with ammonium molybdate and ascorbic acid at pH 4.

Reagents

A. *ATP solution* 5×10^{-3}M
B. *Buffer mixture*, pH 8.4:
    1.0 ml 0.1M Tris solution
    1.0 ml 0.1M 2-amino-2-methyl-1,3-propanediol solution
    1.0 ml 0.1M HCl
    0.3 ml 2.2×10^{-2}M $MgCl_2$ solution.
C. *Incubation medium*: 1 volume ATP solution (A) + 1 volume buffer mixture (B).
D. *Molybdate reagent:* 2 ml 2.5% ammoniummolybdate solution, and 46 ml acetate buffer (0.1M acetic acid, 0.065M sodium acetate). Just prior to use add 2 ml 1% ascorbic acid solution. The concentration of the acetate buffer is chosen to adjust the TCA-extract to pH 4–4.1.
E. *Trichloroacetic acid* (TCA) 30%.
F. *Phosphate standard:* 10 μl 0.150M KH_2PO_4 solution + 1.0 ml incubation medium.

Procedure

a. Enzyme assay

(1) Depending on the enzyme activity, incubate 0.01–0.1 μg frozen-dried tissue samples or 0.1–1.0 μl homogenate in 3 × 50-mm micro test tubes with 5 μl incubation medium (C). Incubation time: 30–60 minutes; temperature: 37°C.

(2) Stop enzyme reaction with 1 μl TCA (ice cold) and keep test tubes in ice bath. Mix with vibrator and centrifuge.

(3) Transfer 5 μl supernatant into 3 × 50-mm micro test tube and add 50 μl molybdate reagent (D). Mix and allow to stand at room temperature for 15–30 minutes. Read absorbance in a 10-mm microcuvette at 870 nm (or nearby wavelength) against water. The small volume requires careful adjustment of the

microcuvettes in the vertical position. This is not possible with all instruments (see page 12). If the reading requires more than 50 μl in the cuvette, all volumes and the amounts of tissue have to be at least doubled.

b. Phosphate standard: incubate 5 μl phosphate standard (F) and proceed as with enzyme assay (2–3).

c. Reagent blank: incubate 5 μl incubation medium (C) and proceed as with enzyme assay (2–3). If the enzyme activity is determined in homogenates, a corresponding volume of redistilled water is added to (b) and (c).

Calculation

The calculation is based on the phosphate standard. The reagent blank (c) is subtracted from (a) and (b). The enzyme activity is expressed in μmoles phosphate/min. $\times$ g dry weight.

ALKALINE PHOSPHATASE

Principle

Alkaline phosphatase hydrolyzes *p*-nitrophenylphosphate. *p*-Nitrophenol liberated is determined colorimetrically.

Reagents

A. *Incubation medium*:
   5.0 ml 0.5M aminomethylpropanediol buffer, pH 10.0
   0.250 ml 0.1M *p*-nitrophenylphosphate solution
   0.025 ml 10% bovine serum albumin solution
   0.010 ml 1.0M $MgCl_2$ solution
   Stored frozen, the solution is stable for about one week.

B. *NaOH* 0.1N

C. *p-Nitrophenol standard*:
   4 μl 1×10^{-2}M *p*-nitrophenol solution + 100 μl incubation medium.

Procedure

a. Enzyme assay
   (1) Depending on the enzyme activity, incubate 0.01–0.1 μg frozen-dried tissue samples or 0.1–0.5 μl homogenate in 3 × 50-mm micro test tubes with 3 μl incubation medium (A). Incubation time: 30–60 minutes; temperature: 37°C.
   (2) Stop enzyme reaction with 50 μl NaOH (B). Mix with vibrator and centrifuge.
   (3) Read absorbance in 10-mm microcuvettes at 400–410 nm against water. The small final volume requires careful adjustment of the microcuvettes in the vertical position. This is not possible with all instruments (see page 12). If the reading requires more than 50 μl in the cuvette, all volumes and the amounts of tissue have to be at least doubled.

b. *p*-Nitrophenol standard: incubate 3 μl standard (C) and proceed as with enzyme assay (2–3).

c. Reagent blank: incubate 3 μl incubation medium (A) and proceed as with enzyme assay (2–3). If the enzyme activity is determined in homogenates, a corresponding volume of redistilled water is added to (b) and (c).

Calculation

The calculation is based on the *p*-nitrophenol standard. The reagent blank (c) is subtracted from (a) and (b), The enzyme activity is expressed in μmoles/min. × g dry weight.

Acid phosphatase

To assay acid phosphatase, the same procedure is used. The aminomethylpropanediol buffer is replaced by acetate buffer, pH 5.4, 0.2M. Since the substrate is unstable in acid solution, the incubation medium has to be prepared fresh every day.

CARBONIC ANHYDRASE (CA)

Literature: Roughton, R. J. W., and V. H. Booth, Biochem. J. **40**, 319 (1946). Mattenheimer, H., and H. DeBruin, Anal. Biochem. **4**, 222 (1962) (ultramicromethod).

Principle

When CO_2 is dissolved in water, it is hydrated to H_2CO_3

$$CO_2 + H_2O \rightleftharpoons H^+ + HCO_3^-$$

CA accelerated this reaction equally in both directions. The difference between the spontaneous hydration of CO_2 and the hydration in the presence of the enzyme is used as a measure of the activity. CO_2-saturated water is added to a weak Veronal buffer, pH 8.0, containing Bromthymol Blue. The time it takes for the pH to drop to 6.3 is measured.

Equipment

1. Micro test tubes: 50 mm long and 2 mm inside diameter, internally coated with silicone. The freshly coated tubes are heated at 150°C for at least 2 hours.
2. Constriction pipets: 300 μl, 230 μl, 12 μl, 8 μl, and a double constriction pipet of 9 μl. Glass or polyethylene constriction pipets may be used. Exceptions to this are the 8-μl pipet, which is used to pipet CO_2-saturated water, and the double constriction pipet. The latter is easier to make from polyethylene than from glass.
3. Incubation unit, consisting of an ice bath, vibrator connected to a powerstat and a holder for two test tubes, a 100-ml polyethylene bottle, a stirrer, and a CO_2 (100%) tank (see Figure 35).
4. Ice bath with rack for microtest tubes
5. Stopwatch.

Reagents

A. *Veronal*, 0.022M
B. *Veronal sodium*, 0.22M
C. *Veronal/veronal-Na buffer*, 0.02M, pH 8.0: 10 ml (A) + 1.1 ml (B). Check pH and adjust if necessary.
D. *Bromthymol Blue*, 0.2% in 50% ethanol
E. *Redistilled water* with 11.8 mg peptone per 100 ml (Bacto-peptone, Difco Laboratories)

F. *Redistilled water* saturated with CO_2 at O°C (= 0.071 M CO_2)
G. *Phosphate buffer*, 0.02M, pH 6.3
H. *Incubation medium:* mix 300 μl buffer (C), 230 μl aqueous peptone solution (E) and 12 μl indicator (D).
I. *Color standard*: made up as (H), but with phosphate buffer (G) instead of Veronal buffer (C).

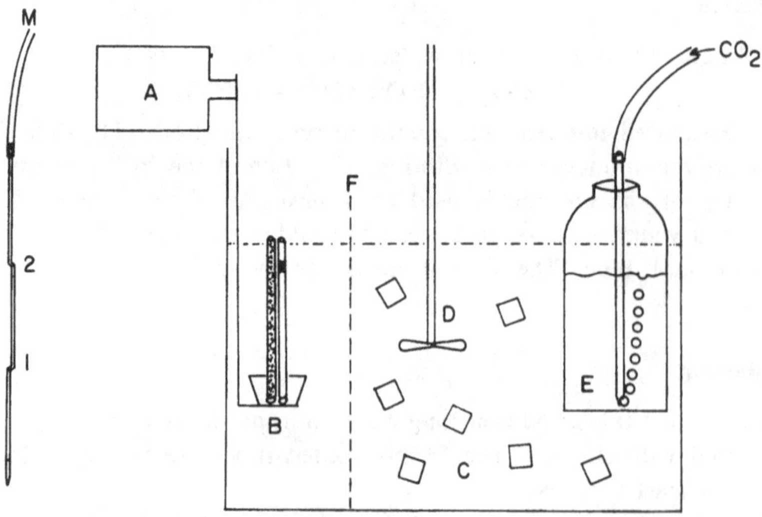

Figure 35. Determination of carbonic anhydrase activity.
Left: polyethylene double-constriction pipet. The volume between 1 and 2 is 9 μl. M = mouth tube.
Right: incubation unit: (A) vibrator connected to a powerstat; (B) holder for 2 micro test tubes, made from a rubber stopper; (C) ice bath; (D) stirrer; (E) polyethylene bottle for CO_2-saturated water; (F) wire screen, to keep ice away from test tubes.

Procedure

In the upper third of each test tube a seal is formed with incubation medium (H), using the 9 μl double constriction pipet. The pipet is filled with the solution up to constriction 2 (Figure 35). The tip of the pipet is set on the wall of the test tube at the level where the seal is to be formed, and the fluid is delivered slowly by applying slight pressure through the mouth tube, while the test tube is slowly rotated. If more than 9 μl is needed to form the seal, excess fluid can be delivered from the pipet but must be aspirated back to constriction 1 after the seal has formed. A seal is preferable to placing the medium in the bottom of the micro test tube because the color change is easier to see with the uniform diameter of the seal, and mixing by vibration is faster in a seal. One test tube is completely filled with color standard (I). The filled test tubes are then placed in a rack in an ice bath to equilibrate the seal to 0°C. The ultramicromethod was developed to determine the activity of CA in nephron cells dissected from frozen-dried kidney sections. The dry weight of the dissected groups of cells should be between 10 and 150 mμg (weighed on a quartz-fiber balance according to O. H. Lowry). For other tissues the required amount has to be determined individually.

The specimens are introduced into the cold seal with a glass needle under a stereoscopic microscope. If enzyme solutions are used (homogenates, extracts), an aliquot not exceeding 0.3 μl is added to the seal with a constriction pipet. To determine the spontaneous hydration of CO_2, five test tubes are prepared and no tissue sample is added.

In order to determine the carbonic anhydrase activity, a test tube containing the seal with the specimen (or for the blank reaction containing the seal without a specimen) is placed in the holder in the ice bath beside the tube with the color standard (Figure 35). The seal must be well below the water level. CO_2-saturated water is then added to the seal with the 8 μl pipet. This pipet must be kept in the ice cold CO_2 water for if allowed to warm before use, gas bubbles would appear in the pipet, not only blocking it but also leading to a loss of CO_2. The tip of the pipet containing CO_2-saturated water is placed on the glass wall approximately 1 mm above the seal and then emptied quickly by applying pressure through the mouth tube. As soon as the pipet is emptied, the stopwatch is pressed and the vibrator is switched on for not more than 1–2 seconds to mix the solutions. It is important not to exceed this mixing time in order to prevent a loss of CO_2. The vibration intensity has to be adjusted with the powerstat so that thorough mixing is achieved. It is usually necessary to repeat the mixing for 1 second when the color change becomes visible because the color change seems to be somewhat slower at the surface. The time is measured for the color to change to yellowish-green; this can be observed with little difficulty by comparison with the color standard. It is advisable to have a good light source in front of the incubation unit. The time for at least five blank reactions (spontaneous CO_2 hydration) must be measured in addition to the enzyme reaction.

Calculation

t_o = reaction time without enzyme (in seconds)

t = reaction time with enzyme

G = weight of specimen in mμg
U = μmoles CO_2 hydrated per gram dry weight per minute at O°C

$$U = \left(\frac{t_o - t}{t - 1}/G\right) \times 63.18 \times 10^6$$

If volumes and/or concentrations of the reagents deviate from the above, the factor must be recalculated (see original literature). Under the experimental conditions $t_o = 100 \pm 1$ seconds.

Example

Cells from proximal convoluted tubules dissected from human kidney = 30 mμg; $t_0 = 100$; $t = 91$

$$U = \left(\frac{100\text{–}91}{90}/30\right) \times 63.18 \times 10^6 = 210390\ \mu\text{moles/g} \times \text{min.}$$

The coefficient of variation of the method is about ±10%. For familiarization with this technique, the use of a commercial CA preparation of which a dilution series is prepared is recommended. 0.2–0.3 μl are used for the activity determination. By plotting activity versus concentration, a straight line is obtained up to t_o–t = 60.

PROTEIN (with Folin's phenol reagent)

Literature: Lowry, O. H., N. J. Rosebrough, A. L. Farr, and R. J. Randall, J. Biol. Chem. **193**, 265 (1951) (modified).

Principle

Tyrosine and trytophan in proteins react with Folin's phenol reagent to give a blue color which is read photometrically. The color intensity varies somewhat with different proteins because of the disparity in their tyrosine and tryptophan content. But the method is extremely sensitive and can be recommended for enzyme work, especially when absolute values are not required.

Reagents

A. *NaOH* 1.0N

B. Solution of 2% *sodium carbonate* (anhydrous) and 0.02% *sodium* or *potassium tartrate*

C. *Copper sulfate solution* 0.5% ($CuSO_4 \times 5\,H_2O$)

D. Mix 50 vol. (B) with 1 vol. (C). Prepare fresh every day.

E. *Phenol reagent according to Folin Ciocalteu* with an acid concentration of 1.0N. The acidity of the commercial reagent (Fisher) is approximately 2N. Titrate an aliquot with NaOH against phenolphthalein and dilute the reagent accordingly.

F. *Trichloroacetic acid* 10%

G. *Protein standard*: a mixed human serum is recommended to plot a standard curve. The serum protein concentration is in turn determined against bovine serum albumin (BSA); 1.00 mg BSA = 0.97 mg human serum protein. BSA itself is not a suitable protein working standard because it tends to surface denaturation in dilute solutions.

For the protein standard curve the human serum is diluted to 5–50 mg protein/100 ml. The standard curve should be periodically verified. In addition it is recommended that a serum standard be included in each series of determinations. If the measured value deviates from the theoretical value, a new standard curve must be constructed with the currently used reagents.

Procedure

a) Dilute protein solution to 0.2–5 μg/10 μl (= 2–50 mg/100 ml)
b) Tissue samples should have a dry weight of 0.4 to 5 μg.

Method 1: serum and other protein solutions
Pipet into a micro test tube

10 μl protein solution
10 μl NaOH (A)
100 μl reagent (D)

Mix with vibrator and allow to stand for 10 minutes. Hold test tube horizontally and add as a side drop

10 μl reagent (E)

Mix side drop in with vibrator (this step is critical—mixing must be rapid). Allow to stand for at least 30 minutes. Read absorbance in 10-mm microcuvette at 700–750 nm against a blank with water instead of protein solution. Also prepare a standard with 10 μl standard serum. Use the same pipet for unknown, standard and water. If the photometer does not permit reading between 700 and 750 nm, measurements may be made with reduced sensitivity between 550–600 nm.

Method 2: protein precipitated by TCA
Pipet into a micro test tube

10 μl protein solution
10 μl TCA (F)

Mix with vibrator and centrifuge. Aspirate supernatant with a polyethylene pipet with a fine tip (suction pump). Add to the precipitate

10 μl NaOH (A)

Dissolve precipitate by vibration, heat gently if necessary. Then add

10 μl H_2O
100 μl reagent (D)

and proceed as directed in Method 1. Treat protein standard with TCA.

Method 3: dry tissue (frozen-dried tissue sections or frozen-dried homogenate)
Pipet into a micro test tube

10 μl NaOH (A)

Add tissue specimen with a fine tipped glass needle under a stereoscopic microscope. Mix with vibrator and wait until tissue has dissolved; heat gently if necessary. Then add

10 μl H_2O
100 μl reagent (D)

and proceed as directed in Method 1. The standard contains protein standard instead of H_2O. If less tissue is available, all volumes may be cut in half. The small final volume requires careful vertical adjustment of the microcuvette in the light path. This is not possible with all photometers (see page 12).

Appendixes

Appendix I

Table to convert ΔA = 0.100 into mμmoles NADH (NADPH) at 366 nm, 340 nm and 10-mm light path, for various volumes of the assay mixture

Assay volume μl	mμmoles NADH (NADPH) 366 nm	340 nm	Assay volume μl	mμmoles NADH (NADPH) 366 nm	340 nm
100	3.00	1.60	255	7.65	4.08
105	3.15	1.68	260	7.80	4.16
110	3.30	1.76	265	7.95	4.24
115	3.45	1.84	270	8.10	4.32
120	3.60	1.92	275	8.25	4.40
125	3.75	2.00	280	8.40	4.48
130	3.90	2.08	285	8.55	4.56
135	4.05	2.16	290	8.70	4.64
140	4.20	2.24	295	8.85	4.72
145	4.35	2.32	300	9.00	4.80
150	4.50	2.40	305	9.15	4.88
155	4.65	2.48	310	9.30	4.96
160	4.80	2.56	315	9.45	5.04
165	4.95	2.64	320	9.60	5.12
170	5.10	2.72	325	9.75	5.20
175	5.25	2.80	330	9.90	5.28
180	5.40	2.88	335	10.05	5.36
185	5.55	2.96	340	10.20	5.44
190	5.70	3.04	345	10.35	5.52
195	5.85	3.12	350	10.50	5.60
200	6.00	3.20	355	10.65	5.68
205	6.15	3.28	360	10.80	5.76
210	6.30	3.36	365	10.95	5.84
215	6.45	3.44	370	11.10	5.92
220	6.60	3.52	375	11.25	6.00
225	6.75	3.60	380	11.40	6.08
230	6.90	3.68	385	11.55	6.16
235	7.05	3.76	390	11.70	6.24
240	7.20	3.84	395	11.85	6.32
245	7.35	3.92	400	12.00	6.40
250	7.50	4.00			

Appendix II

Preparations of buffer solutions

Aminomethylpropanediol buffer, 0.05M

A. 0.2M 2-amino-methyl-1,3-propanediol: 21.05 g diluted to 1 liter with redistilled water.

B. 0.2N HCl
50 ml (A) + x ml, (B), diluted with redistilled water to 200 ml.

pH	x	pH	x
7.8	43.5	9.0	16.7
8.0	41.0	9.2	12.5
8.2	37.7	9.4	8.5
8.4	34.0	9.6	5.7
8.6	29.5	9.8	3.7
8.8	22.0	10.0	2.0

Carbonate buffer, 0.05M

A. 0.2M Na_2CO_3: 21.2 g anhydrous Na_2CO_3 diluted to 1 liter with redistilled water.

B. 0.2M $NaHCO_3$: 16.8 g diluted to 1 liter with redistilled water.
x ml (A) + y ml (B), diluted with redistilled water to 200 ml.

pH	x	y	pH	x	y
9.2	4.0	46.0	10.0	27.5	22.5
9.3	7.5	42.5	10.1	30.0	20.0
9.4	9.5	40.5	10.2	33.0	17.0
9.5	13.0	37.0	10.3	35.5	14.5
9.6	16.0	34.0	10.4	38.5	11.5
9.7	19.5	30.5	10.5	40.5	9.5
9.8	22.0	28.0	10.6	42.5	7.5
9.9	25.0	25.0	10.7	45.0	5.0

Collidine buffer 0.05M

A. 0.2M 2,4,6-collidine: 26.4 ml diluted to 1 liter with redistilled water.

B. 0.1N HCl

25 ml (A) + x ml (B), diluted with redistilled water to 100 ml.

The values for x are given for assay temperatures of 23° and 37°C.

pH	x(23°)	x(37°)
6.5	44.0	43.0
6.6	42.5	41.6
6.7	41.2	40.1
6.8	40.8	38.3
6.9	38.0	36.2
7.0	35.5	33.5
7.1	33.2	31.1
7.2	30.5	28.4
7.3	27.5	25.4
7.4	25.0	22.5

pH	x(23°)	x(37°)
7.5	22.3	22.0
7.6	19.3	17.5
7.7	16.6	15.0
7.8	14.1	12.5
7.9	12.0	10.6
8.0	10.0	9.0
8.1	8.6	7.5
8.2	7.2	6.0
8.3	5.8	4.7

Glycine NaOH buffer 0.05M

A. 0.2M glycine

15.01 g diluted to 1 liter with redistilled water

B. 0.2N NaOH

50 ml (A) + x ml (B), diluted with redistilled water to 200 ml.

pH	x
8.6	4.0
8.8	6.0
9.0	8.8
9.2	12.0
9.4	16.8

pH	x
9.6	22.4
9.8	27.2
10.0	32.0
10.4	38.6
10.6	45.5

Phosphate buffer 0.1M

A. 0.1M KH_2PO_4: 13. 51 g diluted to 1 liter with redistilled water.

B. 0.1M Na_2HPO_4: 14.19 g diluted to 1 liter with redistilled water x ml (B) made up with (A) to 100 ml.

pH	x
5.8	8.0
6.0	12.0
6.2	18.5
6.4	26.2
6.6	36.0
6.8	50.0

pH	x
7.0	61.0
7.2	72.0
7.4	80.8
7.6	87.0
7.8	91.5

Triethanolamine buffer, 0.1M

A. 0.1M Triethanolamine hydrochloride: 18.56 g diluted to 1 liter with redistilled water.

B. 0.1N NaOH

x ml (B) made up with (A) to 100 ml.

pH	x	pH	x
7.0	2.75	8.0	12.30
7.2	3.35	8.2	14.40
7.4	5.50	8.4	15.55
7.6	7.65	8.6	17.35
7.8	10.10	8.8	18.60

Tris buffer, 0.1M

A. 0.2M Tris (hydroxymethyl) aminomethane: 24.2 g diluted to 1 liter with redistilled water.

B. 0.2N HCl

50 ml (A) + x ml (B), diluted with redistilled water to 100 ml.

pH	x	pH	x
7.2	44.2	8.2	21.9
7.4	41.4	8.4	16.5
7.6	38.4	8.6	12.4
7.8	32.5	8.8	8.1
8.0	26.8	9.0	5.0

Veronal-Na-HCl buffer, 0.1M

A. 0.2M Veronal-Na: 41.2 g diluted to 1 liter with redistilled water.

B. 0.2 HCl

50 ml (A) + x ml (B), diluted with redistilled water to 100 ml.

pH	x	pH	x
6.8	45.0	8.2	12.5
7.0	43.0	8.4	9.0
7.2	39.0	8.6	6.0
7.4	32.5	8.8	4.0
7.6	27.5	9.0	2.5
7.8	22.5	9.2	1.5
8.0	17.5		

Appendix III

Reagents and Reagent Kits

Reagents, inorganic and organic, must be of analytical grade. Biochemicals—enzymes, coenzymes and substrates—should be of the highest purity available. In our laboratory we use biochemical reagents from Boehringer Mannheim Corporation, New York; E. Merck (EM-Reagents Division, Brinkmann Instruments, Westbury, New York); Sigma Chemical Company, St. Louis, Missouri; Calbiochem, Los Angeles, California; Mann Research Laboratories, New York; Schwarz Bioresearch, Inc., Orangeburg, New York; General Biochemicals, Chagrin Falls, Ohio. This should not imply that biochemicals of other manufacturers are not to be recommended, but we have no experience with these products.

It is in the nature of some biochemicals to deteriorate easily. Therefore, most biochemical reagents must be stored at +4°C.

Reagent kits for chemical and enzymatic analyses, and especially for enzyme determinations, have become available in increasing numbers. If these test kits are used for micromethods, one must be aware that the procedures described in this book may differ from the methods of the test kits. The latter methods can in most cases be adapted to the microscale by a proportional reduction of all volumes; the corresponding micromethod in this book may serve as a guide.

Precaution is necessary with some enzyme preparations which may contain other enzymes as impurities. When an enzyme is used in a coupled test to catalyze an auxiliary or indicator reaction, it is essential to have exact information on contaminants and to make the necessary corrections by including a "reagent-enzyme" blank; see the example on page 136: GOT content of MDH-preparations used in the assay of GOT activity.

Appendix IV

Simplified Tests in Clinical Chemistry

Literature: Adams, E. C., Jr., and H. Mattenheimer, Z. Klin. Chem. 3, 1 (1965).

In the past 15 years a new type of test was developed to qualitatively, and with some tests semiquantitatively, analyze urine and other body fluids for a variety of substances.

TEST STICKS

Test sticks are strips of filter paper impregnated with all reagents necessary for the respective test. The stick is dipped into the solution to be analyzed; a color develops in one minute or less, and the result is obtained by comparison with a color chart.

TEST TABLETS

The reagents are combined in a tablet, which is either moistened with or dissolved in the solution to be tested.

The tests described in the following paragraphs are those developed and marketed by Ames Company, Inc., Elkhart, Indiana. The products of other manufacturers are listed in the literature cited above.

Detection of glucose in urine

Clinistix (stick test): the test depends on the following reactions:

$$\text{Glucose} + O_2 \xrightarrow{\text{glucose oxidase}} H_2O_2 + \text{gluconolactone}$$

$$H_2O_2 + o\text{-tolidine} \xrightarrow{\text{peroxidase}} \text{blue color}$$

The test stick is impregnated with the enzymes, chromogen, a background red dye and buffers. The stick is dipped into urine and after 10 seconds the color is compared to a color chart. The sensitivity of this enzyme test generally exceeds that of reduction tests. Depending on a combination of variable factors in urine, such as specific gravity, pH, and the amount of inhibitors, such as ascorbic acid, the sensitivity ranges from 10^{-2} to 10^{-1} g per 100 ml urine. Since so many variable factors influence the enzyme reactions, the test does not quantitate glucose in urine. High concentrations of ascorbic acid in urine will inhibit the oxidation-reduction reaction and give false negative answers.

Clinitest (tablet test): a copper reduction test; its essential ingredients are cupric sulfate, citric acid, sodium hydroxide and sodium carbonate. The reaction may be represented by the following equation:

$$Cu^{++} + \text{sugar} \xrightarrow[\text{alkali}]{\text{heat}} \underset{\substack{\text{green or}\\\text{orange color}}}{Cu_2O} + \text{glyconic acid} + \text{other degradation products}$$

The necessary heat is generated by the reaction of citric acid and water with sodium hydroxide. In the recommended method five drops of urine are added to ten drops of water in a special test tube provided with the kit. The tablet is added (the solution boils); 15 seconds after boiling ceases the tube is shaken and the color compared to the chart which has colors for negative, trace, $\frac{1}{4}$, $\frac{1}{2}$, 1 and 2% sugar. It is necessary to observe the tube during boiling because in urines containing more than 2% sugar the solution will pass through orange to a color that resembles the one for 3/4% on the chart. For urines containing more than 2% sugar, it is recommended that two drops of urine be diluted with 13 drops distilled water; the result is then multiplied by 2.5.

Protein in urine

Albustix (stick test): the test is based on the protein error of acid-base indicators. Certain pH indicators, in the presence of protein, will have a color indicating a higher or lower pH than the actual value in the solution determined with a pH-meter. The color change at constant pH is proportional to the amount of protein present.

The stick contains Tetrabromphenol Blue as the indicator and citrate buffer to maintain the pH at 3. The indicator changes from yellow to green and finally to blue in the presence of protein. The stick is dipped into the urine and the color that develops is compared to a color chart with values of negative, trace, 30, 100, 300 and more than 1000 mg protein per 100 ml.

Blood in urine and feces

All chemical tests for occult blood depend on the ability of hemoglobin to catalyze the peroxide oxidation of certain indicators such as *o*-tolidine, benzidine, guaiac and others. Most tests use hydrogen peroxide or an organic peroxide that will release hydrogen peroxide in aqueous solution.

Occultest (tablet test): the test tablets are composed of strontium peroxide, *o*-tolidine, calcium acetate, tartaric acid, sodium bicarbonate and tabletting ingredients. The reaction may be represented by the following equations:

$$SrO_2 + 2H_2O \longrightarrow H_2O_2 + Sr(OH)_2$$

$$H_2O_2 + o\text{-tolidine} \xrightarrow{\text{hemoglobin}} \text{blue color}$$

The test is run by putting a drop of urine on a square of filter paper, placing a tablet on the square, and then adding to the tablet two drops of water with a five second interval, so the water extracts the reagents and runs off the tablet onto the filter paper. After two minutes the blue color developing around the tablet is compared to a color chart. The intensity of the color developed after two minutes and the rate of color development are both related to the amount of blood present. Generally the *Occultest* will detect 1 μl of blood per 50–100 ml of urine.

Hematest (tablet test): this test is similar to *Occultest* but less sensitive. For testing of feces a thin line smear is made on a filter paper square. The tablet is placed on the smear and two drops of water at an interval of five seconds are allowed to flow over the tablet. A blue color developing on the paper within two minutes indicates the presence of blood.

Hemastix (stick test): the paper strips are impregnated with *o*-tolidine, cumene hydroperoxide, wetting agents, color enhancers and buffers. The reaction may be represented as

$$ROOH + o\text{-tolidine} \xrightarrow{\text{hemoglobin}} \text{blue color}$$

The stick is dipped into the urine and after one minute its color is compared to a chart which has colors corresponding to small, moderate and large amounts of blood. Hemastix appears to be about as sensitive as Occultest.

Cumene hydroperoxide and similar organic hydroperoxides are much more specific for the hemoglobin peroxidase reaction than for the leukocyte peroxidase reaction. Thus urines containing only white cells will not react with Hemastix. The blood peroxidase tests react not only with hemoglobin but also with myoglobin.

The test detects free hemoglobin and hemoglobin released from erythrocytes on contact with the stick. Thus there is no correlation between the erythrocyte count in urine and the intensity of the color on the stick. Erythrocytes are hemolyzed when standing in hypo- and hypertonic urine, but even freshly voided urine may contain free hemoglobin in addition to red blood cells. It is assumed that some erythrocytes are destroyed during passage through the nephron. Occultest and Hemastix will of course detect free hemoglobin and myoglobin in hemoglobinuria and myoglobinuria.

Combined tests

Uristix (stick test): the tests for glucose and protein are combined on one stick. The protein zone on the tip of the stick and the glucose zone above are separated by an impervious barrier. The composition of the zones is essentially the same as described for *Clinistix* and *Albustix*.

Hemacombistix (stick test): this is a four-zone stick. Urinary glucose, protein, hemoglobin and pH can be determined simultaneously. The composition of the zones is essentially the same as for *Clinistix, Albustix* and *Hemastix*.

Detection of ketone bodies in urine

Acetest (tablet test): the tablet contains sodium nitroprusside, glycine and phosphate buffer. To perform this test a drop of urine is placed on the tablet surface; a purple color on the tablet indicates the presence of acetoacetate or acetone.

Ketostix (stick test): the cellulose strip contains sodium nitroprusside, glycine and buffer. When the strip is dipped into urine containing ketone bodies, a purple color will develop within 15 seconds. Ketostix and Acetest will detect 5–10 mg acetoacetate per 100 ml urine.

Bilirubin in urine

Ictotest (tablet test): two principles are involved in this test. A special filter paper adsorbs and concentrates bilirubin while a stabilized diazonium salt couples with bilirubin to produce a purple color. In the procedure five drops of urine are placed on the filter paper; the tablet is placed over the urine spot and moistened with two drops of water. If bilirubin is present, a purple color develops around the tablet. The tablet contains *p*-nitrobenzenediazo-*p*-toluene sulfonate and sulfosalicylic acid. The test is very sensitive and picks up 0.1 mg bilirubin per 100 ml.

Phenylketonuria

Phenistix (stick test): phenylpyruvic acid reacts with ferric ions to produce a green to blue-grey color. *Phenistix* is a paper strip impregnated with ferric ions, magnesium ions to counteract phosphate inhibition and cyclohexamic acid to provide the proper pH. A blue-grey color develops when a stick is dipped into a urine containing phenylpyruvic acid.

Drug metabolites in urine

Phenistix can also be used to detect a variety of drug metabolites that react with ferric ions. The colors resulting from these reactions are different from the color obtained with phenylpyruvic acid, and confusion is not possible. For instance, Phenistix reacts with the metabolites of *p*-amino-salicylate to give a red color and with salicylates to give a purple color.

Cystinuria

Cystine in urine can be detected by a combination of Acetest with cyanide reduction. A tablet of Acetest is placed in the well of a white procelain spot plate and moistened with a drop of alkaline cyanide (1% sodium cyanide in 1N NaOH); a drop of urine is added. If cystine is present, a cherry color forms around the tablet within one minute. Under these conditions ketone bodies do not produce a color with Acetest.

Application of the simplified tests to blood and serum

The number of simplified tests for substances in blood or serum is much smaller than those for urine. The main reason is that the difference between normal and abnormal values is less in blood. Simplified tests for substances in blood offer the most promising area for further development.

Of the tests described for urine, Acetest and Ketostix can be used for the detection of ketone bodies, and Phenistix for the detection of salicylates in blood or serum. For serum, Ketostix is the most useful as it can be dipped into the serum and the stick color compared to the color chart after 15 seconds. Ketostix will detect 5–10 mg acetoacetic acid in 100 ml serum. With Acetest, a thin smear of serum is placed on a paper, a tablet is then placed on top of the still moist smear and left for 30 seconds. The tablet is inverted and the color observed. For whole blood Acetest can be used. A drop of blood is placed on the tablet; when the blood clots, the clot is lifted off and a purple color is observed.

Salicylate in blood can be detected with Phenistix. A purple color indicates the presence of salicylate. To detect salicylate intoxication in infants, the following combination of testing urine and serum for salicylates has been suggested: if the urine is negative, a salicylate intoxication can be ruled out. If the urine is positive, serum should be tested. A negative test in serum rules out intoxication, while a positive test in all probability indicates salicylate intoxication.

Determination of glucose in blood

Dextrostix (stick test): this test was especially developed to determine glucose in blood. The filter paper strips are impregnated with glucose oxidase, peroxidase and an indicator system. A semipermeable membrane holds back protein and cells. In the procedure a drop of capillary blood is placed on the reagent zone of the stick. After exactly one minute, the blood is washed off with a sharp stream of water from a wash bottle. Immediately after rinsing, the color is compared to a color chart with color shades for the following concentrations: 40–65–90–130–150–200–250 mg per 100 ml blood.

The simplified tests can be performed at the bed side or in the office, and they serve as screening tests. It is well, however, to be familiar with the limitations of a particular test and not to demand more of it than it can do. The physician may frequently be able to decide from the result of one of the simple tests whether or not a urine or serum sample should be sent to the laboratory for quantitative analysis.

Index

D

E

F

G

H

I

Printed and Bound in the U.S.A.
LithoCrafters, Inc., Ann Arbor, Michigan